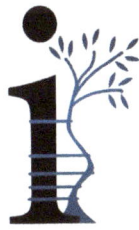

QUESTIONS AND ANSWERS FOR

BACK PAIN SUFFERERS

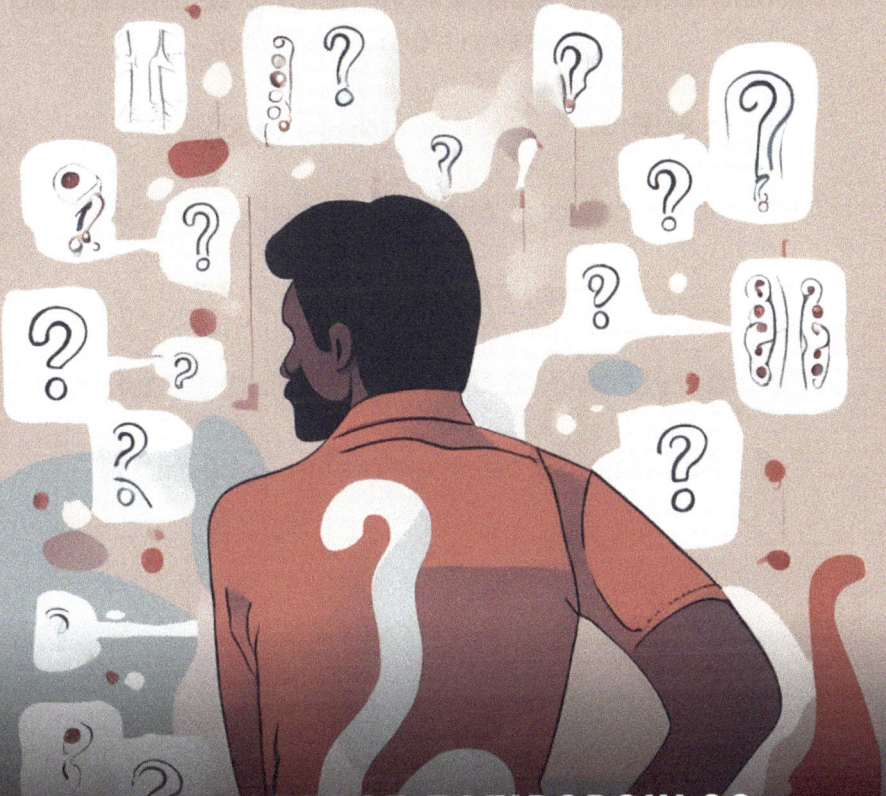

PROF. GEORGE ZAFIROPOULOS

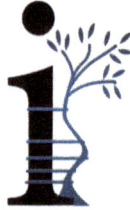

Copyright © George Zafiropoulos

Author: George Zafiropoulos @2024

Title: Questions and Answers for Back Pain Sufferers

ISBN: 978-1-0686737-7-1

Category: Pain Management / Health / Back Pain

Publisher: Breakfree Forever Publishing

IMPORTANT NOTICES / DISCLAIMERS

The depicted experience may be considered as not typical. Your background, education, experience and work ethic may differ. This is used as an example and not a guarantee of success. Individuals do not track the typicality of its student's experiences. Your results may vary.

The contents of this training, such as text, graphics, images, and other material are intended for informational and educational purposes and not for the purpose of rendering medical or mental health advice. The contents of this training are not intended to substitute for professional medical advice, diagnosis, and/or treatment. Please consult your medical professional before making changes to your diet, exercise routine, medical regimen. lifestyle, and or mental health care.

This is not a medical consultation or medical advice. This is a guide to be followed, aiming to improve the quality of your life. You can keep all necessary and relevant material for you and discard what is not working for you.

Stories shared during the sessions of the modules are true experiences of me personally or patients with whom I have crossed paths during consultations over the years and no personal details are shared within the course that can make them identifiable to anybody.

CONTENTS

INTRODUCTION

In this book, I will attempt to answer questions that may be commonly asked by diverse groups of people. These questions are based on the subject that was analysed in other books the author created, and their purpose is to specifically be used for educational purposes. The information is not and will not be represented as a replacement for an expert medical opinion that is the result of a meticulous clinical examination, but only as indicative educational material in an attempt to guide back pain sufferers in the management of their back problems.

The questions are the result of frequent inquiries expressed by different groups of people. It may be noticed that in some cases, some answers have similar content. This is because the same or similar question was asked, or the question belongs to a different category of people. The explanations are as brief as possible and act as a framework, giving different thoughts to the readers. More information about the subjects can be found in other books by the same author or in the plethora of other books and publications on this subject matter.

Who am I and what makes me qualified to talk about back pain?

I studied Medicine. I specialised and became a Consultant Orthopaedic Surgeon. During my career, I have seen and treated a vast number of people who have suffered from back pain, so I have a great understanding of the condition, the implications, limitations, and effects of it on people's lives. I have a total of over 43 years in Medicine, Science, and Experience on my side, and 39 of those years within Orthopaedic surgery. I observed the struggles different groups were going through due to long chronic back pain issues and the great difficulties they had. I saw their inability to talk about their pain and ask for help, either at a personal or social level. The reluctance to ask for help in their working environment or the "bullying" they experienced from other people in their jobs or their social life. This is the reason I decided to write the present information.

I would be humbled if you would allow me to share these questions and try to answer, in a brief way, the potential questions you have. The answers are based on years of experience and research. I wish to point out that this is only for guidance, and it is not a medical consultation.

This must be performed by your own medical practitioner. The material is only here to assist your understanding of what low back pain is and how it is affecting us on multiple levels and systems of our body. The created material will guide us through different pathways, and step by step, we will find together the solution.

This is not a medical consultation, but it is an adventure through the cold corridors of science and the tumultuous ways of the mind, as both body and mind suffer the same from this condition.

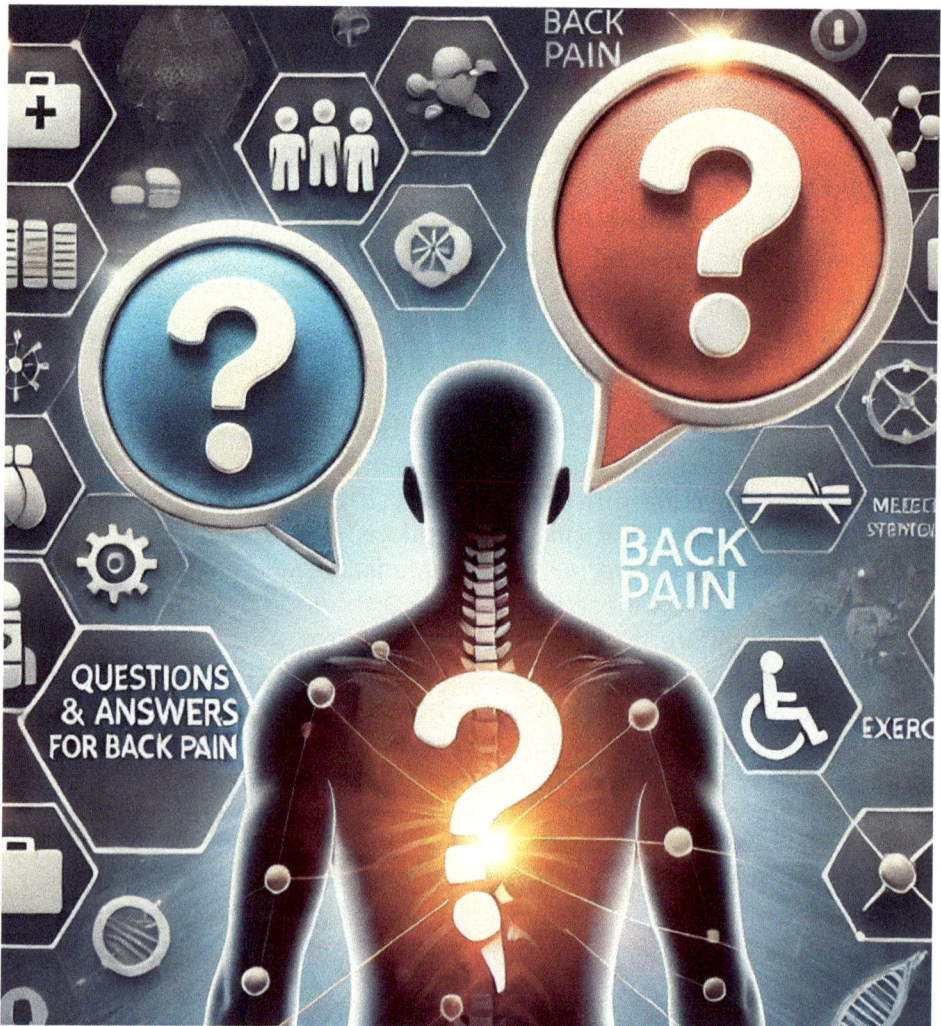

GENERAL QUESTIONS ABOUT BACK PAIN

These questions reflect the concerns and uncertainties people with back pain often have, ranging from understanding the cause of their pain to finding effective treatment options.

WHAT COULD BE CAUSING MY BACK PAIN?

Back pain can be caused by a variety of factors, including:

Muscle or Ligament Strain:
Overexertion, heavy lifting, or sudden awkward movements can strain the muscles and ligaments in your back, leading to pain.

Herniated or Bulging Discs:
The discs in your spine can bulge or rupture, pressing on nerves and causing pain.

Degenerative Disc Disease:
As you age, the discs in your spine can wear down, leading to pain.

Arthritis:
Osteoarthritis can affect the joints in your spine, causing pain and stiffness.

Skeletal Irregularities:
Conditions like scoliosis (curvature of the spine) can lead to back pain.

Osteoporosis:
This condition weakens bones, making them more brittle and prone to fractures, which can cause back pain.

Spinal Stenosis:
A narrowing of the spinal canal can put pressure on the spinal cord and nerves, leading to pain.

Poor Posture:
Long-term poor posture can strain your spine and lead to pain.

Infections or Tumours:
Although rare, infections or tumours in the spine can cause back pain.

Psychological Factors:
Stress, anxiety, and depression can contribute to or exacerbate back pain.

Understanding the underlying cause of your back pain is important for determining the appropriate treatment and management strategies but these strategies must be conducted under the direct guidance of specialised health professionals.

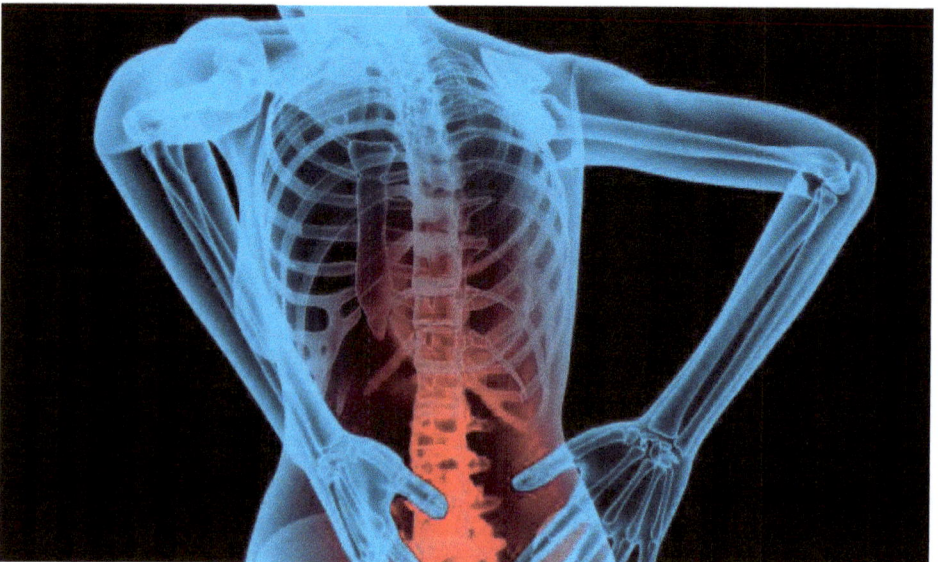

WHAT TREATMENTS ARE AVAILABLE TO RELIEVE MY BACK PAIN?

There are a variety of treatments available to help relieve back pain, depending on the underlying cause, severity of pain, and your overall health. Here are some common treatment options:

Medications (Please check with your doctor):

- **Over-the-Counter Pain Relievers:** Medications like Paracetamol or nonsteroidal anti-inflammatory drugs (NSAIDs) can help reduce pain and inflammation.

- **Muscle Relaxants:** These can be prescribed for short-term relief of severe muscle spasms associated with back pain.

- **Prescription Pain Relievers:** For more severe pain, doctors may prescribe stronger painkillers, such as opioids, but these are typically used for short periods due to the risk of dependency.

- **Topical Pain Relievers:** Creams, ointments, or patches containing pain-relieving ingredients can be applied directly to the skin over the painful area.

Physical Therapy:

- **Exercise Programs:** A physical therapist can design a customised exercise plan to strengthen your back and core muscles, improve flexibility, and promote proper posture.

- **Manual Therapy:** Techniques such as spinal manipulation or mobilisation by a physical therapist, chiropractor, or osteopath can help improve spinal alignment and reduce pain.

- **Education:** Physical therapists also teach you proper body mechanics and ergonomic techniques to prevent further injury.

Lifestyle Modifications:

- **Weight Management:** Medications like Paracetamol or nonsteroidal anti-inflammatory drugs (NSAIDs) can help reduce pain and inflammation.

- **Smoking Cessation:** Smoking can impair blood flow to the spine and contribute to disc degeneration, so quitting can help.

- **Posture Correction:** Improving your posture while sitting, standing, and lifting can prevent or alleviate back pain.

Heat and Cold Therapy:

- **Cold Packs:** Applying ice to the affected area can reduce inflammation and numb the pain.

- **Heat Therapy:** Heat pads, warm baths, or heating wraps can relax tense muscles and increase blood flow to the affected area, promoting healing.

Alternative Therapies:

- **Acupuncture:** This traditional Chinese medicine technique involves inserting thin needles into specific points on the body to relieve pain.

- **Chiropractic Care:** Chiropractors use hands-on spinal manipulation to help alleviate pain and improve function.

- **Yoga and Pilates:** These practices can improve flexibility, strength, and posture, contributing to back pain relief.

Injections:

- **Corticosteroid Injections:** These injections can reduce inflammation and provide pain relief, especially for conditions like sciatica or herniated discs.

- **Nerve Blocks:** : These are used to block pain signals from specific nerves and can be diagnostic as well as therapeutic.

Surgical Treatments:

- **Discectomy:** Removal of part of a herniated disc that is pressing on a nerve.

- **Laminectomy:** Removal of part of the vertebra to relieve pressure on the spinal cord or nerves.

- **Spinal Fusion:** Joining two or more vertebrae together to stabilise the spine and reduce pain.

- **Minimally Invasive Procedures:** Procedures like vertebroplasty or kyphoplasty can stabilise fractured vertebrae.

Behavioural Therapy:

- **Cognitive-Behavioural Therapy:** It can help manage chronic pain by changing negative thought patterns and improving coping strategies.

Assistive Devices:

- **Braces and Supports:** Wearing a back brace can provide support and relieve pain, particularly during recovery from an injury.

Relaxation Techniques:

- **Mindfulness and Meditation:** These practices can help reduce stress, which can exacerbate back pain, and improve your ability to manage pain.

It is important to consult with a healthcare provider to determine the most appropriate treatment plan for your specific condition.

In many cases, a combination of these treatments may be recommended to achieve the best results.

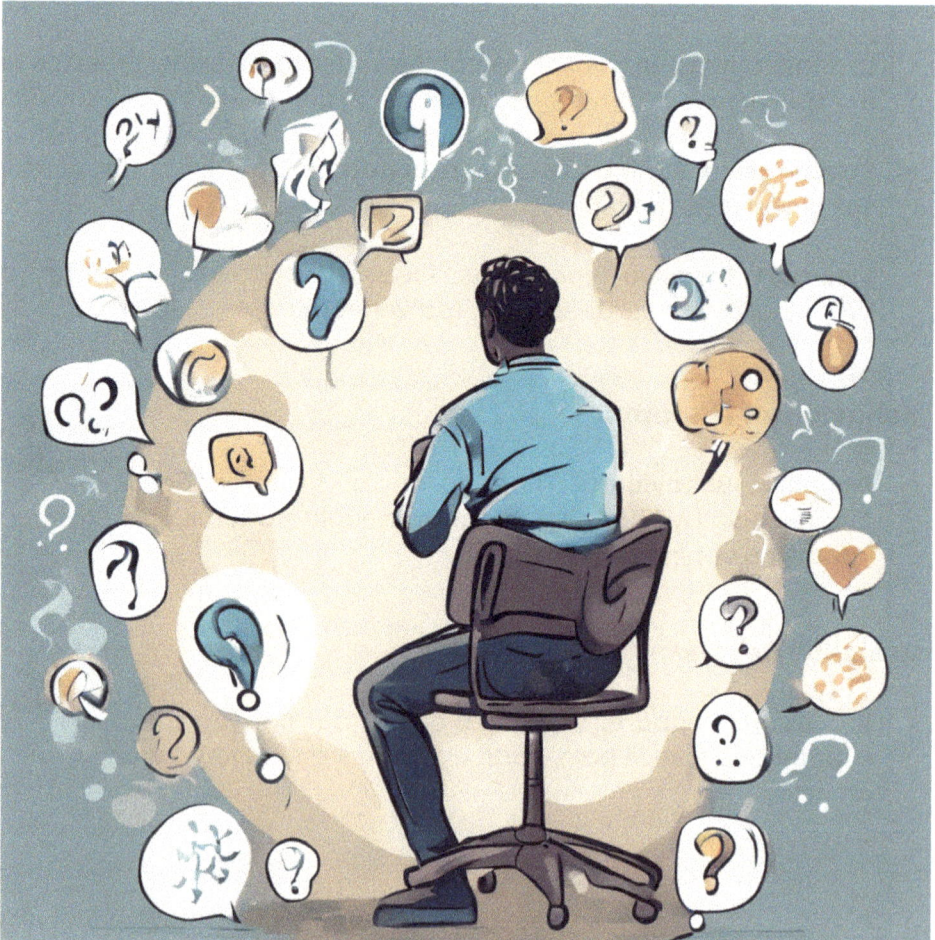

ARE THERE ANY EXERCISES OR STRETCHES THAT CAN HELP ALLEVIATE MY BACK PAIN?

There are several exercises and stretches that can help alleviate back pain by strengthening the muscles that support your spine, improving flexibility, and reducing tension. However, it's important to consult with a healthcare provider or physical therapist before starting any new exercise routine, especially if you have a specific condition or injury.

Pelvic Tilts:

- Purpose: Strengthens the abdominal muscles and helps stretch the lower back.

- How to Do It:

  - Lie on your back with your knees bent and feet flat on the floor.

  - Tighten your abdominal muscles, flattening your lower back against the floor.

  - Hold for 5-10 seconds, then relax.

  - Repeat 10-15 times.

Knee-to-Chest Stretch:

- Purpose: Stretches the lower back and relieves tension.

- How to do It:

  - Lie on your back with your knees bent and feet flat on the floor.

  - Bring one knee to your chest, keeping the other foot on the floor.

  - Hold for 15-30 seconds, then lower your leg.

  - Repeat with the other leg.

  - Repeat 2-3 times with each leg.

Cat-Cow Stretch:

- Purpose: Improves flexibility in the spine and reduces tension.

- How to Do It:

  - Start on your hands and knees, with your wrists directly under your shoulders and knees under your hips.

  - Inhale and arch your back (Cow Pose), dropping your belly toward the floor and lifting your head and tailbone.

  - Exhale and round your back (Cat Pose), tucking your chin to your chest and drawing your belly button toward your spine.

  - Continue alternating between Cat and Cow for 1-2 minutes.

Child's Pose:

- Purpose: Gently stretches the lower back, hips, and thighs.

- How to Do It:

  - Start on your hands and knees.

  - Sit back onto your heels, reaching your arms forward and lowering your chest toward the floor.

  - Hold for 30 seconds to 1 minute.

  - Breathe deeply and relax into the stretch.

Bridge Exercise:

- Purpose: Strengthens the lower back, glutes, and core muscles.

- How to Do It:

  - Lie on your back with your knees bent and feet flat on the floor, hip-width apart.

  - Tighten your abdominal muscles and lift your hips toward the ceiling, forming a straight line from your shoulders to your knees.

  - Hold for a few seconds, then lower your hips back down.

  - Repeat 10-15 times.

Seated Forward Bend:

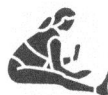

- Purpose: Stretches the lower back and hamstrings.

- How to Do It:

  - Sit on the floor with your legs extended straight in front of you.

  - Reach forward toward your toes, keeping your back straight.

  - Hold the stretch for 15-30 seconds, then release.

  - Repeat 2-3 times.

Bird-Dog Exercise:

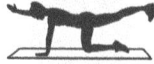

- Purpose: Strengthens the lower back and core muscles.

- How to Do It:

  - Start on your hands and knees, with your wrists directly under your shoulders and knees under your hips.

  - Extend your right arm forward and your left leg straight back, keeping your hips level.

  - Hold for a few seconds, then return to the starting position.

  - Repeat on the opposite side.

  - Perform 10-15 repetitions on each side.

Hamstring Stretch:

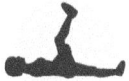

- Purpose: Stretches the hamstrings, which can help relieve tension in the lower back.

- How to Do It:

  - Lie on your back with one leg extended straight on the floor.

  - Lift the other leg toward the ceiling, holding behind the thigh or calf.

  - Keep the leg straight and gently pull it toward you until you feel a stretch.

  - Hold for 15-30 seconds, then switch legs.

  - Repeat 2-3 times per leg.

Piriformis Stretch:

- Purpose: Stretches the piriformis muscle, which can help alleviate sciatica-related back pain.

- How to Do It:

  - Lie on your back with both knees bent.

  - Cross one leg over the other, placing the ankle on the opposite knee.

  - Gently pull the uncrossed leg toward your chest, feeling a stretch in the buttock of the crossed leg.

  - Hold for 15-30 seconds, then switch legs.

  - Repeat 2-3 times per leg.

Wall Sits:

- Purpose: Strengthens the back, legs and core muscles.

- How to Do It:

  - Stand with your back against a wall, feet shoulder-width apart.

  - Slowly slide down the wall until your knees are bent at about a 90-degree angle.

  - Hold the position for 10-15 seconds, then slide back up the wall.

  - Repeat 8-10 times.

Incorporating these exercises and stretches into your daily routine can help alleviate back pain and improve your overall spinal health. Remember to perform each movement slowly and with control and stop if you experience any pain.

IS IT SAFE TO CONTINUE MY USUAL ACTIVITIES, OR SHOULD I REST MORE?

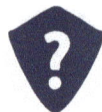

Deciding whether to continue your usual activities or rest more when experiencing back pain depends on the nature and severity of your pain, as well as the activities you are considering. Here are some general guidelines to help you make the right decision:

When to Continue Usual Activities:

- **Mild to Moderate Pain**

  - If your back pain is mild to moderate and not caused by a serious condition, it is generally safe and beneficial to continue with most of your usual activities.

  - Staying active can help maintain flexibility, strength, and overall health, and it can prevent your muscles from becoming stiff and weak.

- **Gradual Resumption**

  - If you've recently experienced a flare-up, you may need to modify your activities temporarily. Gradually return to your normal routine as your pain subsides.

  - Activities like walking, gentle stretching, and light housework are often encouraged as they help keep your muscles engaged without causing undue strain.

- **Benefits of Activity**

  - Movement increases blood flow to the affected area, which can aid in the healing process.

  - Regular physical activity can also help prevent future episodes of back pain by strengthening the muscles that support your spine.

When to Modify or Limit Activities:

- **Severe Pain or Acute Injury**

  - If your back pain is severe, sharp, or the result of an acute injury (e.g. from lifting something heavy or a fall), you may need to temporarily limit your activities.

  - Avoid activities that aggravate your pain, especially those that involve heavy lifting, twisting, or bending.

- **Pain with Specific Movements**

  - If you notice that certain movements or activities consistently worsen your back pain, it may be wise to avoid or modify those activities until you have fully recovered.

- **Signs to Rest**

  - If your pain is accompanied by other symptoms, such as numbness, tingling, or weakness in your legs, or if it interferes with your ability to perform daily tasks, resting and consulting a healthcare provider is recommended.

  - Resting for a day or two may be beneficial in the acute phase, especially if the pain is intense or if you've just experienced an injury.

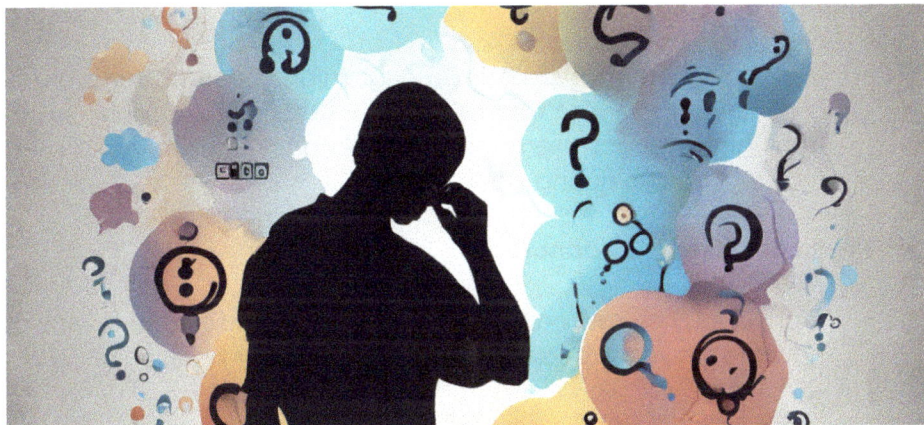

The Role of Rest:

- **Short-Term Rest**

  - Short periods of rest, such as lying down for a few hours or overnight, can help reduce inflammation and allow your body to recover from acute pain or injury.

  - However, prolonged bed rest is generally not recommended, as it can lead to muscle stiffness, weakness, and prolonged recovery times.

- **Active Rest**

  - Instead of complete bed rest, consider "active rest" where you remain as active as possible without causing pain. This might involve gentle movements, short walks, and avoiding positions that exacerbate your pain.

Balancing Activity and Rest:

- **Listen to Your Body**

  - Pay attention to how your body responds to different activities. If something causes pain, modify it or take a break. If you feel better after moving, continue with light activities.

- **Modify Your Routine**

  - Depending on your pain level, you might need to temporarily modify your exercise routine or work tasks. For example, switch from high-impact exercises to low-impact ones, or take more frequent breaks during work.

- **Physical Therapy Guidance:**

  - A physical therapist can provide specific exercises and advice on how to safely stay active while managing your back pain.

General Rule:

Listen your Body.

Continue with Caution: In most cases, it is safe and beneficial to continue with your usual activities, if they do not exacerbate your pain. Movement is often key to recovery.

Modify if Needed: If certain activities cause pain or discomfort, consider modifying or temporarily avoiding them. Gradually resume these activities as your pain improves.

Consult a Professional: If you are unsure about which activities are safe, or if your pain is severe or persistent, it's a good idea to consult with a healthcare provider for specific advice.

The goal is to maintain a balance between staying active and allowing your body the rest it needs to heal. Avoiding prolonged inactivity is advisable, as movement can often aid in recovery and prevent future back issues.

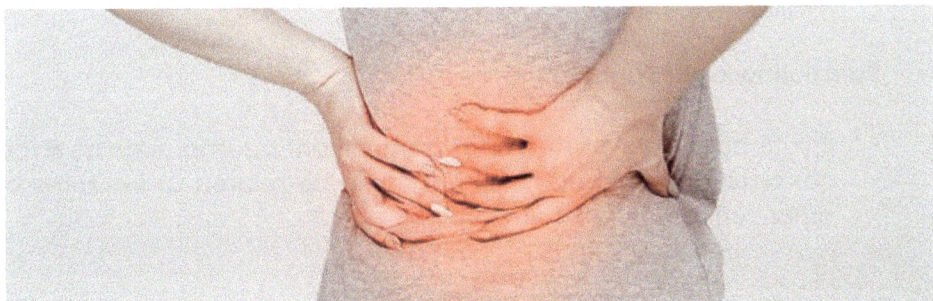

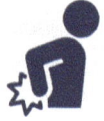

COULD MY BACK PAIN BE A SIGN OF A MORE SERIOUS UNDERLYING CONDITION? (RED OR POTENTIAL RED FLAGS)

While most back pain is due to common, less serious issues such as muscle strain, poor posture, or degenerative changes related to aging, it can sometimes be a sign of a more serious underlying condition.

It's important to be aware of certain symptoms and risk factors that may indicate your back pain is related to a more serious issue.

Persistent or Severe Pain:

- **Mild to Moderate Pain**

  - If your back pain is severe, persistent, and does not improve with rest or over the counter pain medications, it may warrant further investigation.

- **Pain Accompanied by Neurological Symptoms:**

  - If your back pain is accompanied by symptoms such as numbness, tingling, or weakness in your legs, feet, or groin area, it could indicate nerve compression or damage, such as from a herniated disc or spinal stenosis.

  - Loss of bladder or bowel control can be a sign of cauda equina syndrome, a rare but serious condition that requires immediate medical attention.

- **Pain Following Trauma**

  - If your back pain started after a significant trauma, such as a fall, car accident, or sports injury, it could be related to fractures or other serious injuries to the spine.

- **Pain Accompanied by Unexplained Weight Loss:**

    - Unintended weight loss along with back pain could be a sign of a more serious condition, such as an infection, cancer, or other systemic illness.

- **Pain with Fever or Other Signs of Infection:**

    - Back pain accompanied by fever, chills, or night sweats may suggest an infection, such as osteomyelitis (a bone infection) or discitis (an infection of the intervertebral discs).

- **Pain That Worsens at Night:**

    - If your back pain is worse at night or while lying down, and not relieved by rest, it may be indicative of a more serious condition, such as a tumour or spinal infection.

- **History of Cancer:**

    - If you have a history of cancer and develop new or unexplained back pain, it is important to consult a doctor. Back pain could be a sign of metastatic cancer, where the cancer has spread to the spine.

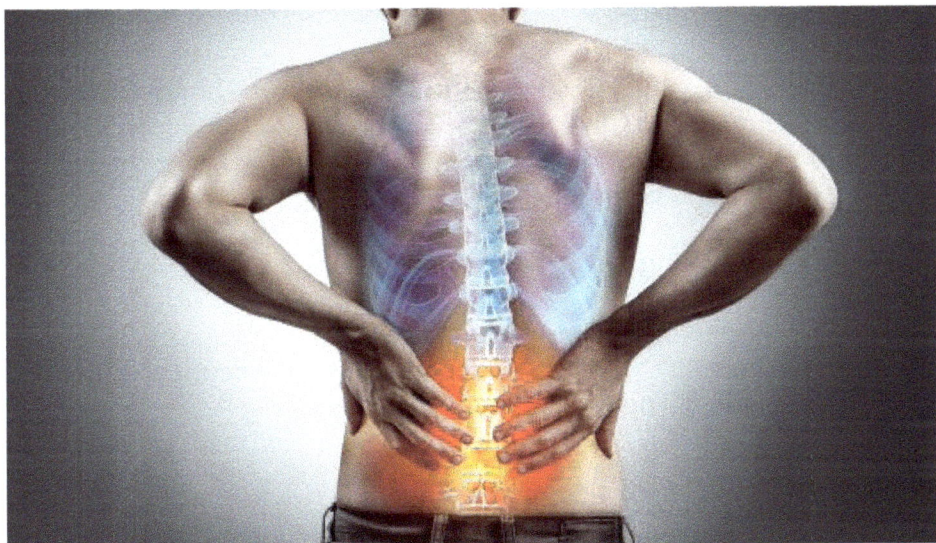

- **Osteoporosis or Risk Factors for Bone Loss:**

  - Individuals with osteoporosis or other risk factors for bone loss are at increased risk for spinal fractures, which can cause severe back pain.

  - However, prolonged bed rest is generally not recommended, as it can lead to muscle stiffness, weakness, and prolonged recovery times.

- **Pain That Radiates to the Abdomen:**

  - If your back pain radiates to the abdomen or chest, it could be related to conditions such as aortic aneurysm or pancreatitis, which require immediate medical attention.

- **Age and Underlying Health Conditions:**

  - Older adults and individuals with underlying health conditions, such as diabetes, immunosuppression, or chronic steroid use, are at higher risk for serious conditions that could cause back pain.

What to Do If You Suspect a Serious Condition:

- **Seek Medical Attention:**

  - If you experience any of the above symptoms or have concerns about your back pain, it's important to seek medical evaluation promptly. Early diagnosis and treatment are crucial for managing serious conditions effectively.

- **Diagnostic Testing:**

  - Your healthcare provider may recommend diagnostic tests such as X-rays, MRI, CT scans, blood tests, or bone scans to determine the cause of your pain.

- **Follow-Up Care:**

  - If your back pain is related to a serious underlying condition, your doctor will develop a treatment plan tailored to your specific diagnosis, which may include medications, physical therapy, or in some cases, surgery.

Summarising it is necessary to say that while back pain is often due to less serious causes, it can sometimes be a sign of a more serious underlying condition.

Being aware of the red flags and seeking medical advice when necessary is important for your health. The red flags warrant further investigation, such as imaging or specialist referral, to rule out serious conditions like infections, fractures, tumours, or neurological disorders. If any of these red flags are present, it is important to seek medical attention promptly. If you are concerned about your back pain, and especially if it is accompanied by other worrying symptoms, it's best to consult a healthcare provider for a thorough evaluation and appropriate care.

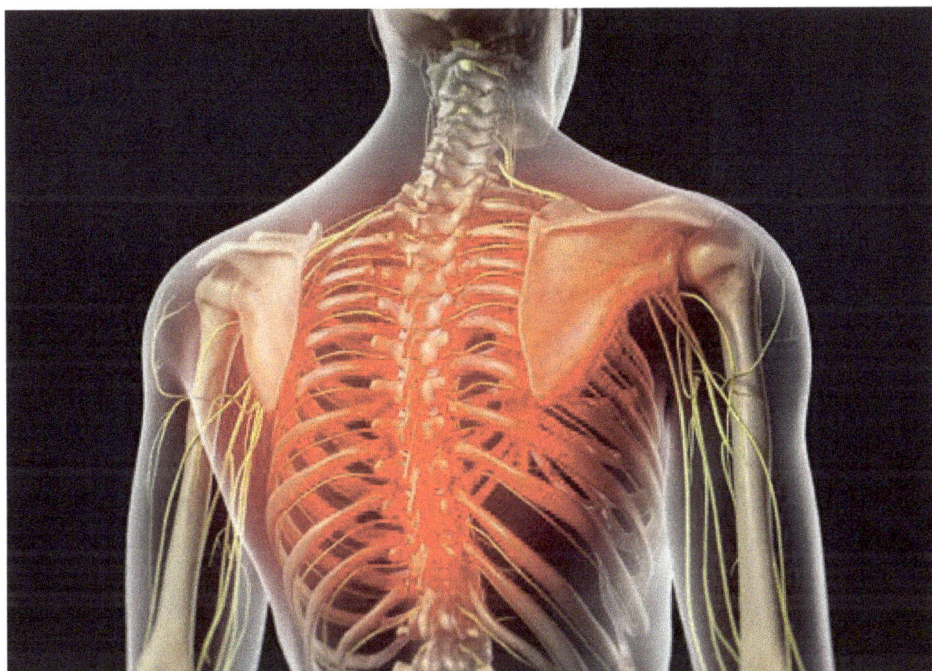

WHAT CAN I DO TO PREVENT MY BACK PAIN FROM COMING BACK?

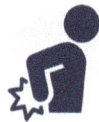

Preventing back pain from recurring involves a combination of lifestyle changes, proper body mechanics, and regular exercises. By adopting healthy habits and being mindful of how you move and take care of your body, you can significantly reduce the risk of future back pain episodes. Here are some strategies to help prevent back pain from coming back:

Persistent or Severe Pain:

- **Why It Matters:** Excess weight, especially around the midsection, can put extra stress on your lower back and contribute to pain.

- **What to Do:** Maintain a healthy weight through a balanced diet and regular exercise. Focus on consuming nutrient-dense foods and avoid excessive calorie intake.

Exercise Regularly:

- **Why It Matters:** Regular physical activity strengthens the muscles that support your spine, improves flexibility, and promotes overall spinal health.

- **What to Do:**

- **Strengthening Exercises:** Focus on exercises that strengthen your core muscles (abdominals and lower back) to provide better support for your spine.

- **Flexibility Exercises:** Incorporate stretching exercises to maintain flexibility in your back, hips, and legs.

- **Low-Impact Aerobic Exercises:** Engage in low-impact activities like walking, swimming, or cycling to improve cardiovascular health without putting excessive strain on your back.

Practice Good Posture:

- **Why It Matters:** Poor posture can place unnecessary strain on your spine, leading to back pain over time.

- **What to Do:**

- **While Sitting:** Sit with your back straight, shoulders relaxed, and feet flat on the floor. Use a chair with good lumbar support or place a small pillow behind your lower back.

- **While Standing:** Stand with your weight evenly distributed on both feet, keep your shoulders back, and avoid slouching.

- **While Sleeping:** Use a supportive mattress and sleep in a position that maintains the natural curve of your spine, such as on your back with a pillow under your knees or on your side with a pillow between your knees.

Use Proper Body Mechanics:

- **Why It Matters:** Incorrect lifting or movements can easily lead to back strain or injury.

- **What to Do:**

- **Lifting:** Bend at your knees and hips, not at your waist, when lifting objects. Keep the object close to your body and lift with your legs, not your back.

- **Carrying:** Avoid twisting while carrying heavy objects. Instead, turn your whole body by moving your feet.

- **Reaching:** Use a step stool or ladder to reach objects on high shelves instead of overstretching.

Strengthen Your Core Muscles:

- **Why It Matters:** A strong core provides essential support for your lower back and reduces the risk of injury.

- **What to Do:**

- **Planks:** Hold a plank position for 20-30 seconds, gradually increasing the time as you get stronger.

- **Bird-Dog Exercise:** Extend one arm and the opposite leg while keeping your back straight, then switch sides.

- **Pelvic Tilts:** Lie on your back with knees bent, tighten your abdominal muscles, and tilt your pelvis upward.

Avoid Prolonged Sitting or Standing:

- **Why It Matters:** Staying in one position for too long can strain your back and lead to discomfort.

- **What to Do:**

- **Breaks:** Take regular breaks to move and stretch if you sit or stand for long periods, such as at work.

- **Standing Desks:** If possible, alternate between sitting and standing throughout the day using a standing desk.

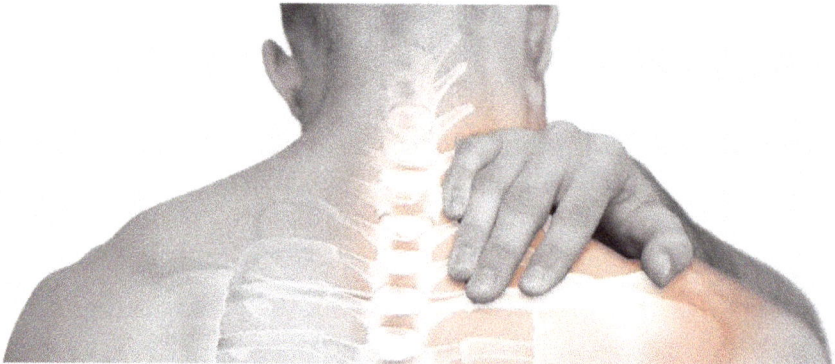

Incorporate Ergonomics into Your Daily Life:

- **Why It Matters:** Proper ergonomics can help prevent strain and injury to your back.

- **What to Do:**

- **Workstation Setup:** Ensure your desk, chair, and computer are set up at the correct height and angle to promote good posture.

- **Supportive Footwear:** Wear shoes that provide good support, especially if you spend a lot of time on your feet.

Quit Smoking:

- **Why It Matters:** Smoking can reduce blood flow to the spine, leading to disc degeneration and back pain.

- **What to Do:** Seek support to quit smoking through counselling, support groups, or smoking cessation programs.

Manage Stress:

Why It Matters: Stress can cause muscle tension and exacerbate back pain.

What to Do:
- **Relaxation Techniques:** Practice stress-relief techniques such as deep breathing, meditation, or yoga.

- **Physical Activity:** Regular exercise can help reduce stress and improve your overall well-being.

Stay Hydrated and Maintain a Healthy Diet:

Why It Matters: Proper hydration keeps your spinal discs healthy, and a balanced diet provides the nutrients needed for strong bones and muscles.

What to Do:
- **Hydration:** Drink plenty of water throughout the day to keep your body hydrated.

- **Diet:** Eat a balanced diet rich in calcium, vitamin D, and other nutrients that support bone health.

Preventing back pain from returning requires a proactive approach that includes regular exercise, proper body mechanics, good posture, and a healthy lifestyle. By making these adjustments, you can significantly reduce your risk of future back pain episodes and maintain a healthy, pain-free back. If you experience recurring back pain despite these efforts, it's important to consult a healthcare provider to explore other potential causes and treatment options.

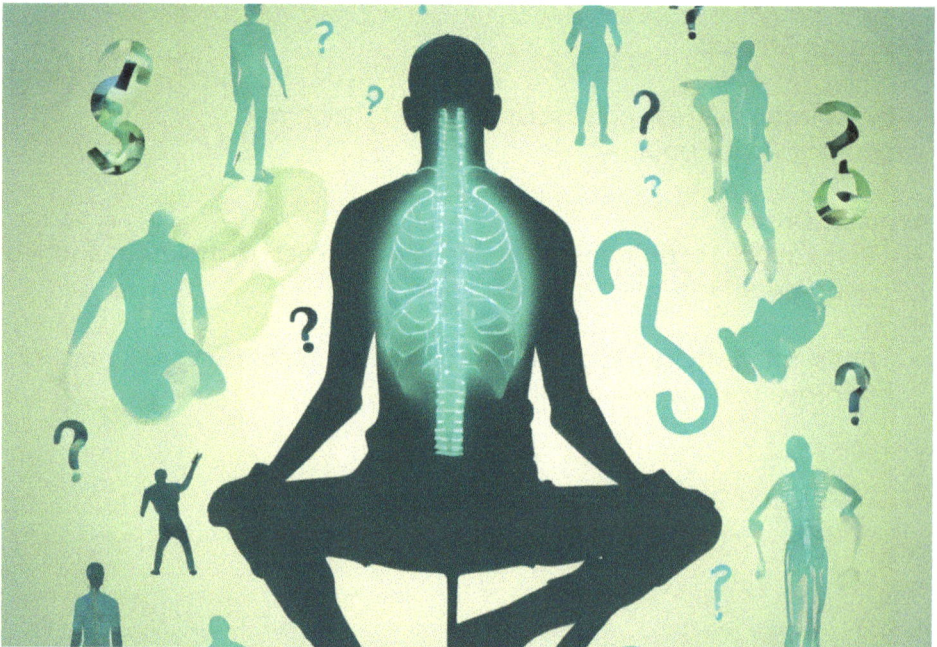

ARE THERE ANY MEDICATIONS OR SUPPLEMENTS THAT CAN HELP WITH BACK PAIN?

There are several medications and supplements that can help manage back pain. The choice of treatment depends on the severity of your pain, the underlying cause, and your overall health. Below is an overview of common medications and supplements that may be beneficial for back pain relief.

Over the Counter for Pain Relief:

Paracetamol: Stress can cause muscle tension and exacerbate back pain.

What to Do:
- **Relaxation Techniques:** Practice stress-relief techniques such as deep breathing, meditation, or yoga.

- **Physical Activity:** Regular exercise can help reduce stress and improve your overall well-being.

Nonsteroidal Anti-Inflammatory Drugs (NSAIDs):

- **How They Work:** NSAIDs reduce inflammation and pain by inhibiting the production of prostaglandins, which are chemicals in the body that cause inflammation.

- **Considerations:** NSAIDs are effective for reducing pain and inflammation, but they can cause stomach upset, ulcers, or kidney problems with long-term use. It's important to take them with food and follow dosing instructions.

Prescription Medications:

Muscle Relaxants:

- **How They Work:** Muscle relaxants help reduce muscle spasms and tension that can contribute to back pain.

- **Considerations:** These medications are typically used for short-term relief and can cause drowsiness, so they should be taken with caution, especially if you need to drive or operate machinery.

Opioids:

- **How They Work:** Opioids are strong pain relievers that work by binding to opioid receptors in the brain to reduce the perception of pain.

- **Considerations:** Opioids are reserved for severe pain that does not respond to other treatments. They carry a risk of addiction, tolerance, and side effects such as constipation, drowsiness, and respiratory depression. They should be used only under close supervision by a healthcare provider.

Antidepressants:

- **How They Work:** Certain antidepressants can help relieve chronic pain by affecting neurotransmitters in the brain that influence pain perception.

- **Considerations:** These medications are often used for chronic pain, especially when associated with conditions like fibromyalgia or nerve pain. They can cause side effects such as dry mouth, drowsiness, or weight gain.

For Topical Pain Relief:

- **How They Work:** Topical treatments are applied directly to the skin over the painful area and work by reducing local inflammation, blocking nerve signals, or desensitising pain receptors.

- **Considerations:** Topical treatments can be a good option for localised pain relief with fewer systemic side effects compared to oral medications.

Corticosteroid Injections:

- **How They Work:** Corticosteroids are powerful anti-inflammatory medications that can be injected directly into the area around the spinal nerves to reduce inflammation and pain.

- **Considerations:** Injections are usually reserved for severe pain, such as from a herniated disc or spinal stenosis. They can provide significant relief but are typically limited to a few treatments per year due to potential side effects like weakened bones and increased blood sugar levels.

Supplements for Back Pain and Musculoskeletal Pain:

Glucosamine and Chondroitin

- **How They Work:** These supplements are thought to support cartilage health and reduce joint pain, including in the spine.

- **Considerations:** Research on their effectiveness is mixed, but some people report relief from chronic joint pain with long-term use. They are generally safe but may interact with blood-thinning medications.

Turmeric (Curcumin):

- **How It Works:** Turmeric contains curcumin, a compound with anti-inflammatory properties that may help reduce pain and inflammation.

- **Considerations:** Turmeric is safe, but it can cause digestive upset in some people. It has blood thinning properties, so need to be taken with care. It's best absorbed when taken with black pepper or fat.

Omega-3 Fatty Acids:

- **How They Work:** Omega-3s have anti-inflammatory effects that may help reduce chronic inflammation and pain in the body, including back pain.

- **Considerations:** Found in fish oil and flaxseed oil, omega-3 supplements are safe but can thin the blood, so they should be used with caution if you are on blood-thinning medications.

Vitamin D:

- **How It Works:** Vitamin D is important for bone health, and deficiency has been linked to chronic pain, including back pain and thinning of bones.

- **Considerations:** If you have low levels of vitamin D, supplementing may help reduce pain. It is important to get your levels checked and to take vitamin D as recommended by your healthcare provider.

Magnesium:

- **How It Works:** Magnesium plays a role in muscle function and relaxation, and deficiency can lead to muscle cramps and spasms, which may contribute to back pain.

- **Considerations:** Magnesium supplements can be beneficial if you are deficient, but too much can cause diarrhoea. It is important to take the appropriate dose.

Remember that Medications and Supplements can play a role in managing back pain, but it is important to use them appropriately and under the guidance of a healthcare provider. Over-the-counter pain relievers, muscle relaxants, and topical treatments can provide relief for many people. Prescription medications, including opioids and corticosteroid injections, are typically reserved for more severe cases. Supplements like glucosamine, turmeric, and omega-3s may offer additional support, particularly for chronic pain.

Always discuss any new medications or supplements with your healthcare provider, especially if you have underlying health conditions or are taking other medications, to ensure they are safe and appropriate for your situation.

GENERAL QUESTIONS ABOUT MANAGEMENT OF BACK PAIN

These questions reflect the practical concerns and strategies that individuals with back pain often consider in the attempt to manage their condition effectively over the long term.

WHAT LIFESTYLE CHANGES CAN I MAKE TO BETTER MANAGE MY BACK PAIN?

Managing back pain often requires a combination of medical treatment and lifestyle changes. Adopting healthier habits and adjusting your daily routine can significantly reduce pain and improve your overall well-being. Here are some lifestyle changes you can make to better manage your back pain:

Maintain a Healthy Weight:

Why It Matters: Carrying excess weight, particularly around the abdomen, can put additional strain on your spine and back muscles, leading to or worsening back pain.

What to Do:
- Focus on a balanced diet rich in fruits, vegetables, whole grains, lean proteins, and healthy fats.

- Engage in regular physical activity to help manage your weight. Activities like walking, swimming, and cycling are gentle on the back and can help maintain a healthy weight.

Exercise Regularly

Why It Matters: Regular exercise strengthens the muscles that support your spine, improves flexibility, and helps maintain a healthy weight, all of which can reduce back pain.

What to Do:
- **Strengthening Exercises:** Include exercises that target your core muscles, such as planks, bridges, and pelvic tilts, to provide better support for your spine.

- **Flexibility Exercises:** Practice stretching exercises like yoga or Pilates to improve flexibility and reduce stiffness in your back.

- **Aerobic Exercise:** Engage in low-impact aerobic activities like walking, swimming, or using an elliptical machine to improve cardiovascular health without putting excessive strain on your back.

Practice Good Posture

Why It Matters: Poor posture can place unnecessary stress on your spine, leading to or exacerbating back pain.

What to Do:
- **Sitting:** Sit with your back straight, shoulders relaxed, and feet flat on the floor. Use a chair with good lumbar support or place a small pillow behind your lower back.

- **Standing:** Stand with your weight evenly distributed on both feet, keep your shoulders back, and avoid slouching. If you stand for long periods, shift your weight between your feet and consider using a footrest.

- **Sleeping:** Use a supportive mattress that maintains the natural curve of your spine. Sleep on your back with a pillow under your knees or on your side with a pillow between your knees.

-

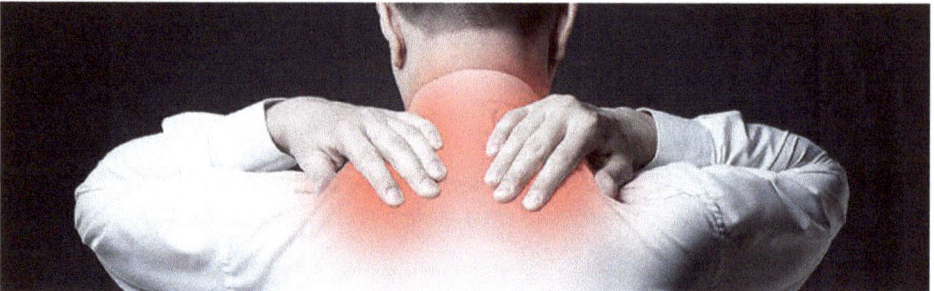

Use Proper Body Mechanics

Why It Matters: Using incorrect techniques for lifting, bending, or twisting can easily strain your back and lead to pain.

What to Do:
- **Lifting:** When lifting heavy objects, bend at your knees and hips, not at your waist. Keep the object close to your body, and lift with your legs, not your back.

- **Carrying:** Avoid twisting your body while carrying heavy objects. Instead, move your feet to turn your whole body.

- **Reaching:** Use a step stool or ladder to reach high objects instead of overstretching or straining your back.

Stay Hydrated

Why It Matters: Proper hydration is important for maintaining the elasticity of the soft tissues in your spine and preventing disc degeneration.

What to Do:
- Drink plenty of water throughout the day. Aim for at least eight cups (about two litres) daily but adjust based on your activity level and climate.

- Limit the intake of dehydrating beverages like alcohol and caffeine.

Quit Smoking

Why It Matters: Smoking impairs blood flow to the spine, which can lead to disc degeneration and increase your risk of developing chronic back pain.

What to Do:
- Seek support to quit smoking, such as counselling, support groups, or smoking cessation programs.

- Consider using nicotine replacement therapy (NRT) or prescription medications to help manage withdrawal symptoms.

Manage Stress

Why It Matters: Stress can cause muscle tension, particularly in the back and neck, and exacerbate pain. Chronic stress can also lead to poor posture and habits that contribute to back pain.

What to Do:
- Practice relaxation techniques such as deep breathing exercises, meditation, or progressive muscle relaxation.

- Engage in regular physical activity, which can help reduce stress and improve your overall mood.

- Consider talking to a therapist or counsellor if stress is significantly impacting your life.

Ergonomics at Work and Home

Why It Matters: Poor ergonomics can lead to strain on your back, especially if you spend long hours sitting or standing in the same position.

What to Do:
- **Workstation Setup:** Ensure that your desk, chair, and computer are set up at the correct height and angle to promote good posture. Use a chair with lumbar support and position your computer screen at eye level.

- **Standing Work:** If you stand for lengthy periods at work, use a cushioned mat to reduce pressure on your spine and legs. Take breaks to sit or stretch.

- **Home Setup:** Apply the same ergonomic principles at home, especially if you work from home or spend significant time sitting or using a computer.

Regular Stretching

Why It Matters: Regular stretching helps maintain flexibility, reduce muscle tension, and prevent stiffness that can contribute to back pain.

What to Do:
- Incorporate daily stretching into your routine, focusing on the back, hamstrings, and hip flexors.

- Try gentle Yoga or Pilates sessions to improve flexibility and strengthen your core muscles.

Stay Active and Avoid Prolonged Sitting

- **Why It Matters:** Prolonged sitting can increase pressure on your lower back and contribute to pain, especially if you sit with poor posture.

- **What to Do:**
- Take regular breaks to stand, stretch, and walk around if you sit for long periods, such as at work or while traveling.

- Consider using a standing desk or alternating between sitting and standing throughout the day.

Summarising the above by Implementing all these lifestyle changes they can help you to better manage your back pain and reduce the likelihood of future episodes. While these adjustments may require some time and effort, the long-term benefits for your spinal health and overall well-being are significant. If you continue to experience back pain despite making these changes, it's important to consult a healthcare provider for further evaluation and personalised advice.

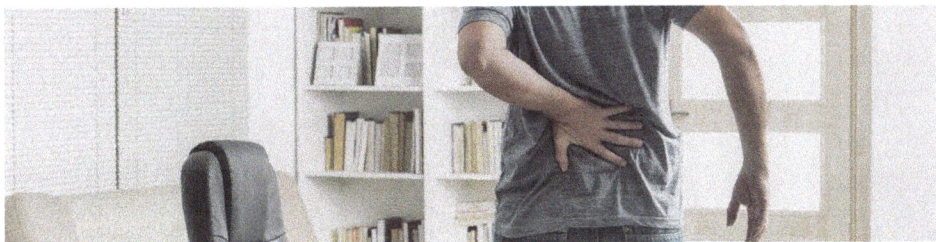

WHAT TYPES OF EXERCISES ARE SAFE AND EFFECTIVE FOR MANAGING MY BACK PAIN?

When managing back pain, it's important to engage in exercises that are safe and effective for strengthening the muscles that support your spine, improving flexibility, and reducing tension. Here is a guide to the types of exercises that are generally recommended for back pain management, along with specific examples of each type.

Core Strengthening Exercises:

Strengthening the core muscles, which include the muscles of the abdomen, back, and pelvis, is essential for providing support to your spine and reducing the risk of back pain.

Exercise Regularly:

- **How to Do It:**

- Lie on your back with your knees bent and feet flat on the floor.

- Tighten your abdominal muscles, flattening your lower back against the floor.

- Hold for 5-10 seconds, then relax.

- Repeat 10-15 times.

Benefits: Strengthens the lower back and abdominal muscles, helping to stabilise the spine.

Bridge Exercise:

- **How to Do It:**

- Lie on your back with your knees bend and feet flat on the floor, hip-width apart.

- Tighten your abdominal muscles and lift your hips toward the ceiling, forming a straight line from your shoulders to your knees.

- Hold for a few seconds, then lower your hips back down.

- Repeat 10-15 times.

Benefits: Strengthens the lower back, glutes, and core muscles.

Bird-Dog Exercise:

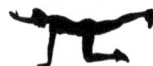

- **How to Do It:**

- Start on your hands and knees, with your wrists directly under your shoulders and knees under your hips.

- Extend your right arm forward and your left leg straight back, keeping your hips level.

- Hold for a few seconds, then return to the starting position.

- Repeat on the opposite side.

- Perform 10-15 repetitions on each side.

Benefits: Strengthens the lower back and core muscles, improving balance and stability.

FLEXIBILITY AND STRETCHING EXERCISES

Stretching exercises help improve the flexibility of the muscles and joints, which can alleviate tension and reduce the risk of injury.

Knee-to-Chest Stretch

- **How to Do It:**

- Lie on your back with your knees bent and feet flat on the floor.

- Bring one knee to your chest, keeping the other foot on the floor.

- Hold for 15-30 seconds, then lower your leg.

- Repeat with the other leg.

- Perform 2-3 times with each leg.

Benefits: Stretches the lower back and relieves tension.

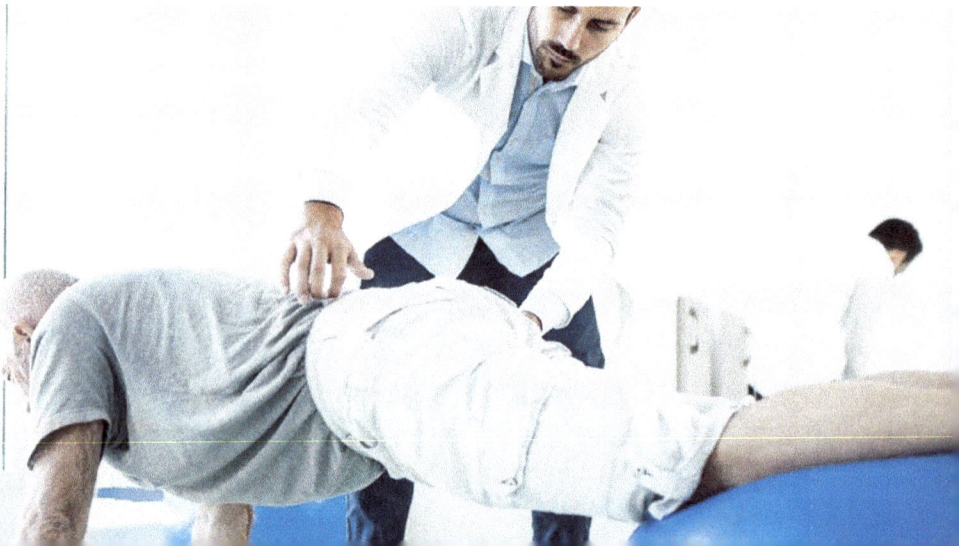

Cat-Cow Stretch:

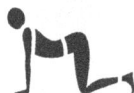

- **How to Do It:**

- Start on your hands and knees, with your wrists directly under your shoulders and knees under your hips.

- Inhale and arch your back (Cow Pose), dropping your belly toward the floor and lifting your head and tailbone.

- Exhale and round your back (Cat Pose), tucking your chin to your chest and drawing your belly button toward your spine.

- Continue alternating between Cat and Cow for 1-2 minutes.

Benefits: Improves flexibility in the spine and reduces tension.

Child's Pose:

- **How to Do It:**

- Start on your hands and knees.
-
- Sit back onto your heels, reaching your arms forward and lowering your chest toward the floor.
-
- Hold for 30 seconds to 1 minute.
-
- Breathe deeply and relax into the stretch.

Benefits: Gently stretches the lower back, hips, and thighs.

LOW-IMPACT AEROBIC EXERCISES

Low-impact aerobic exercises help improve cardiovascular health without putting excessive strain on the back. These exercises also promote overall fitness and weight management, which can reduce the burden on your back.

Walking

- **How to Do It:**

- Aim for 30 minutes of walking at a moderate pace most days of the week.

- Start with shorter walks and gradually increase the duration as your endurance improves.

Benefits: Improves cardiovascular health, strengthens muscles, and supports weight management.

Swimming or Water Therapy

- **How to Do It:**

- Swim laps or participate in water aerobics classes, as the buoyancy of water reduces the impact on your joints and back.

Benefits: Provides a full-body workout that strengthens muscles while minimising strain on the back.

Cycling (Stationary Bike):

- **How to Do It:**

- Use a stationary bike with proper seat adjustment to avoid straining your back.

- Start with short sessions and gradually increase the duration and intensity.

Benefits: Provides a low-impact aerobic workout that improves cardiovascular health without putting pressure on the spine.

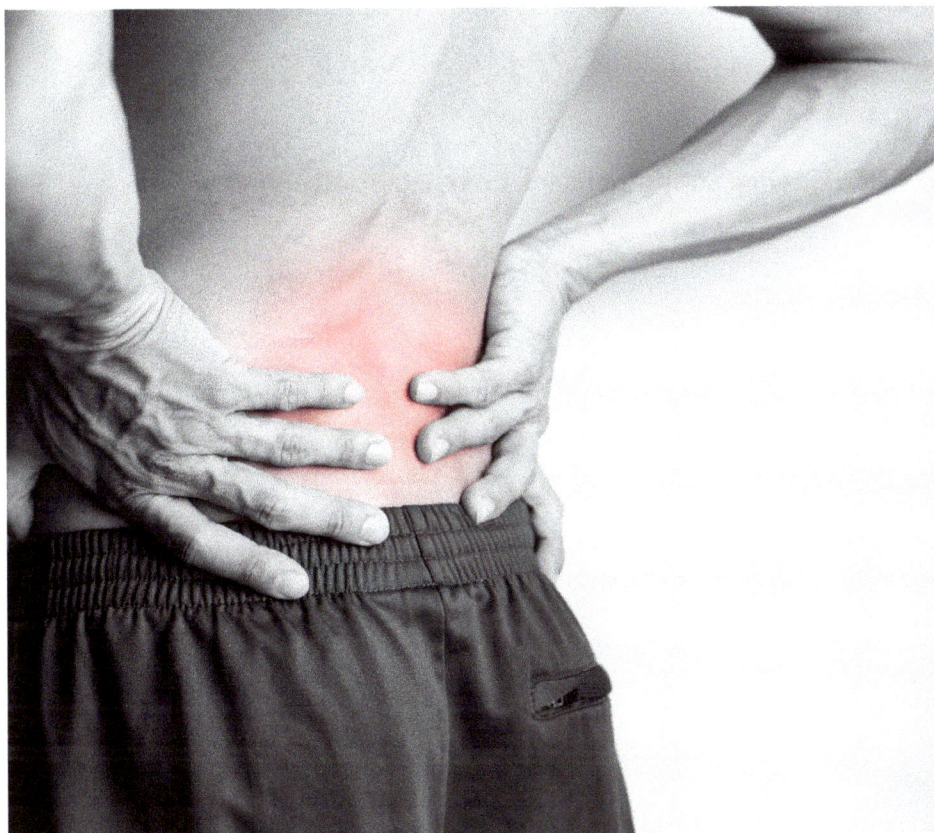

POSTURE AND BALANCE EXERCISES

Improving your posture and balance can help prevent future back pain by making sure that your spine is properly aligned and supported.

Wall Sits

- **How to Do It:**

- Stand with your back against a wall, feet shoulder-width apart.

- Slowly slide down the wall until your knees are bent at about a 90-degree angle.

- Hold the position for 10-15 seconds, then slide back up the wall.

- Repeat 8-10 times.

Benefits: Strengthens the back, legs, and core muscles.

Plank

- **How to Do It:**

- Lie face down with your forearms on the floor and elbows under your shoulders.

- Push up onto your toes and forearms, keeping your body in a straight line from head to heels.

- Hold for 20-30 seconds, then rest.

- Repeat 3-5 times.

Benefits: Strengthens the core muscles and improves stability.

MIND-BODY EXERCISES

Mind-body exercises such as yoga and Pilates focus on flexibility, strength, and relaxation, which can help manage back pain.

Yoga

- **How to Do It:**

- Practice gentle yoga poses that focus on stretching and strengthening the back and core muscles, such as Downward Dog, Cobra, and Cat-Cow.

- Consider joining a yoga class specifically designed for individuals with back pain.

Benefits: Improves flexibility, strength, and posture, and promotes relaxation.

Pilates

- **How to Do It:**

- Engage in Pilates exercises that target the core and back muscles, such as the Hundred, Roll-Up, and Leg Circles.

- Consider taking a Pilates class with an instructor who is knowledgeable about back pain.

Benefits: Strengthens the core muscles, improves posture, and enhances flexibility.

Incorporating these exercises into your routine can help manage back pain, improve your overall spinal health, and prevent future issues. It's important to start slowly and gradually increase the intensity and duration of your exercises as your strength and flexibility improve. Always listen to your body and avoid any movements that cause pain or discomfort. If you're unsure about which exercises are safe for you, or if you have specific concerns about your back pain, consider consulting a physical therapist or healthcare provider for personalised guidance.

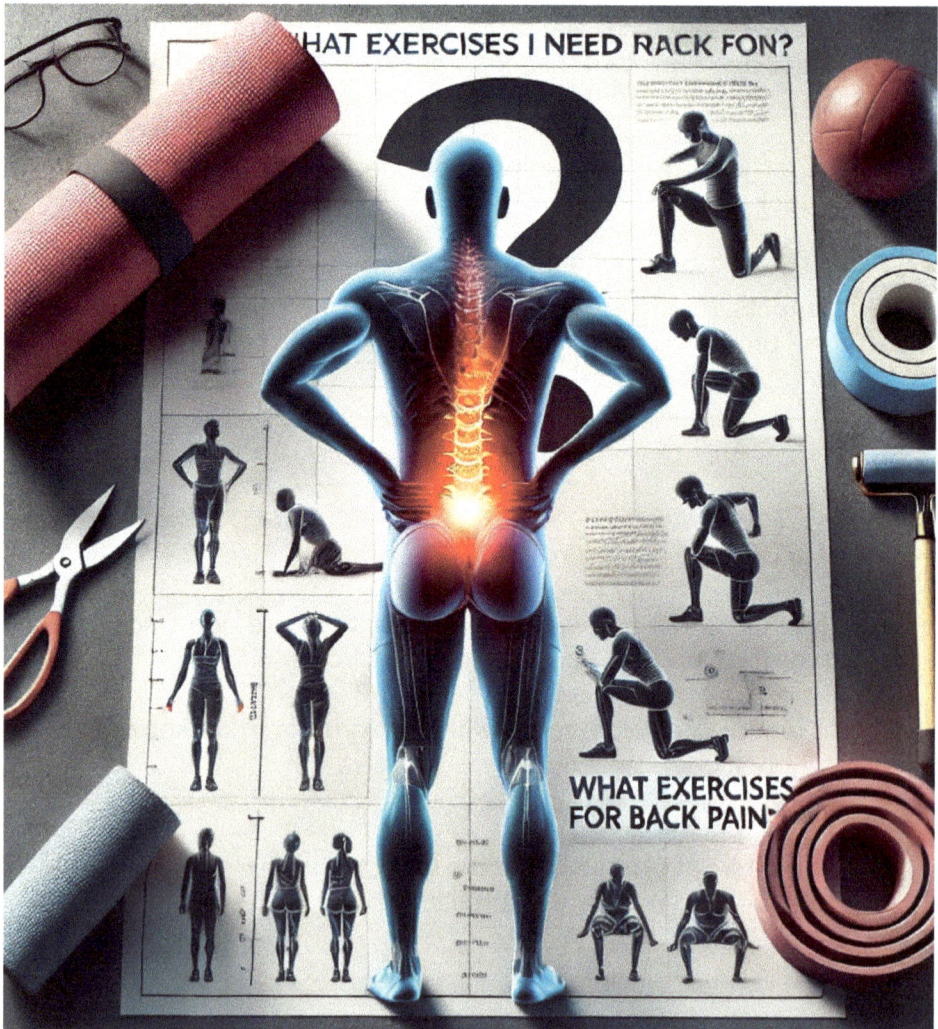

HOW CAN I MODIFY MY WORK ENVIRONMENT OR DAILY ACTIVITIES TO PREVENT FURTHER BACK PAIN?

Modifying your work environment and daily activities is crucial for preventing further back pain, especially if you spend long hours sitting, standing, or engaging in repetitive tasks. By making ergonomic adjustments and being mindful of your posture and movements, you can reduce the strain on your back and minimise the risk of future pain. Here are some strategies to help you modify your work environment and daily activities:

Ergonomic Chair

Why It Matters: A good ergonomic chair provides proper lumbar support and encourages good posture, reducing strain on your lower back.

- **What to Do:**

- Choose a chair with adjustable height, backrest, and armrests.

- Adjust the chair so your feet are flat on the floor, your knees are at a 90-degree angle, and your hips are slightly higher than your knees.

- Use a small pillow or lumbar roll to support the natural curve of your lower back.

Desk Height

Why It Matters: A desk that is too high or too low can cause you to hunch or strain your neck and back.

- **What to Do:**

- Adjust your desk height so your elbows are at a 90-degree angle when typing or using a mouse.

- Keep your keyboard and mouse close enough that you don't have to reach or strain.

Monitor Position

Why It Matters: Placing your monitor at the correct height and distance can prevent neck and upper back strain.

- **What to Do:**

- Position the top of your monitor at or slightly below eye level.

- Place the monitor about an arm's length away from your eyes.

- Use a monitor stand or adjustable desk to achieve the correct height.

Monitor Position

Why It Matters: Placing your monitor at the correct height and distance can prevent neck and upper back strain.

- **What to Do:**

- Position the top of your monitor at or slightly below eye level.

- Place the monitor about an arm's length away from your eyes.

- Use a monitor stand or adjustable desk to achieve the correct height.

Footrest

Why It Matters: If your feet don't comfortably reach the floor, a footrest can help maintain proper posture and reduce strain on your lower back.

- **What to Do:**

Use a footrest if your chair height needs to be adjusted higher for ergonomic reasons, or if your feet don't naturally rest flat on the floor.

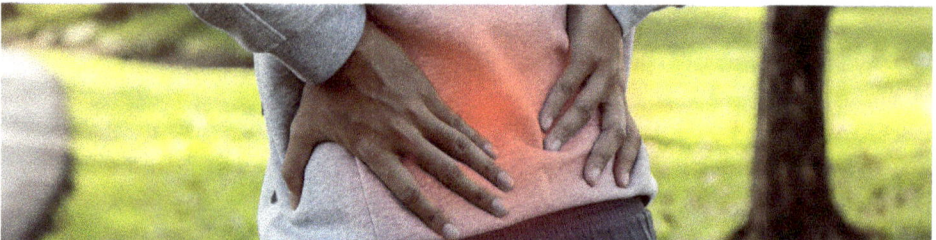

INCORPORATE MOVEMENT INTO YOUR DAY

Mind-body exercises such as yoga and Pilates focus on flexibility, strength, and relaxation, which can help manage back pain.

Frequent Breaks

Why It Matters: Sitting or standing in the same position for extended periods can lead to stiffness and back pain.

- **What to Do:**

- Take short breaks every 30-60 minutes to stand, stretch, and move around.

- Set a timer or use an app to remind you to take breaks throughout the day.

- Consider incorporating quick stretches or walking around your workspace during these breaks.

Alternate Between Sitting and Standing

Why It Matters: Alternating between sitting and standing can reduce the strain on your back and improve circulation.

- **What to Do:**

- Use a sit-stand desk that allows you to change positions throughout the day.

- When standing, shift your weight from one foot to the other or use a footrest to reduce pressure on your lower back.

PRACTICE GOOD POSTURE AND BODY MECHANICS

Sitting Posture

Why It Matters: Maintaining good posture while sitting reduces the strain on your spine and helps prevent back pain.

- **What to Do:**

- Sit with your back straight, shoulders relaxed, and feet flat on the floor.

- Keep your ears aligned with your shoulders and avoid leaning forward or slouching.

- Use a lumbar support cushion to maintain the natural curve of your lower back.

Standing Posture

Why It Matters: Proper standing posture reduces pressure on your spine and helps prevent muscle fatigue.

- **What to Do:**

- Stand with your weight evenly distributed on both feet.

- Keep your shoulders back and your head aligned with your spine.

- Avoid locking your knees, and if standing for long periods, shift your weight periodically.

Lifting Techniques

Why It Matters: Lifting heavy objects, the wrong way is a common cause of back injuries.

- **What to Do:**

- Bend at your knees and hips, not at your waist, when lifting objects.

- Keep the object close to your body and lift with your legs, not your back.

- Avoid twisting your body while lifting; instead, pivot your feet to turn.

ADJUST YOUR DAILY ACTIVITIES

Household Chores

Why It Matters: Activities like vacuuming, gardening, and cleaning can strain your back if not done correctly.

- **What to Do:**

- Use long-handled tools to avoid bending over for extended periods.

- When lifting objects, such as groceries or laundry baskets, use proper lifting techniques.

- Alternate tasks to avoid repetitive strain on the same muscles.

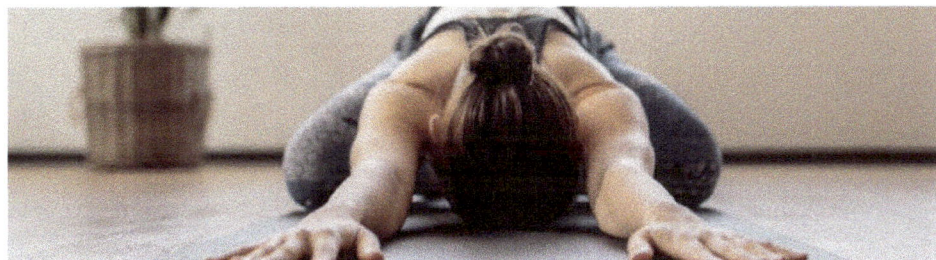

Driving

Why It Matters: Prolonged driving can lead to poor posture and back pain.

- **What to Do:**

- Adjust your car seat to support your lower back and maintain a comfortable posture.

- Use a lumbar roll or cushion if needed.

- Take breaks on long drives to stand, stretch, and move around.

Sleep Environment

Why It Matters: Your sleep position and mattress can affect your back health.

- **What to Do:**

- Choose a mattress that provides adequate support and maintains the natural curve of your spine.

- Sleep on your back with a pillow under your knees, or on your side with a pillow between your knees if you are in pain.

- Avoid sleeping on your stomach, as this can strain your back and neck.

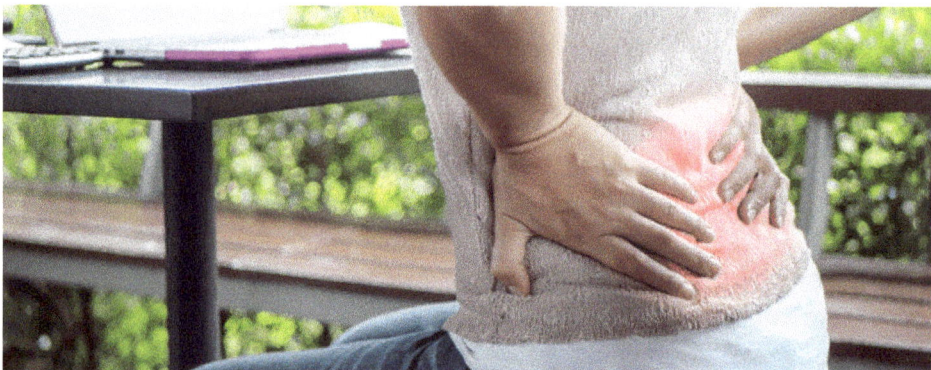

INCORPORATE ERGONOMIC TOOLS AND ACCESSORIES

Ergonomic Accessories

Why It Matters: Ergonomic tools can help reduce strain on your body and improve comfort while working.

- **What to Do:**

- Use an ergonomic keyboard and mouse to reduce strain on your wrists, arms, and shoulders.

- Consider using a headset for phone calls to avoid cradling the phone between your shoulder and ear.

- Use document holders or stands to keep reference materials at eye level.

Supportive Footwear

Why It Matters: Wearing supportive shoes can help maintain good posture and reduce back strain, especially if you spend a lot of time on your feet.

- **What to Do:**

- Choose shoes with good arch support and cushioning.

- Avoid high heels or flat shoes with little support.

- Consider using orthotic inserts if needed for additional support.

By making these modifications to your work environment and daily activities, you can reduce the risk of further back pain and improve your overall comfort and well-being. These changes may require some initial adjustments, but the long-term benefits for your back health are well worth the effort. If you continue to experience back pain despite making these modifications, it's important to consult a healthcare provider for further evaluation and advice.

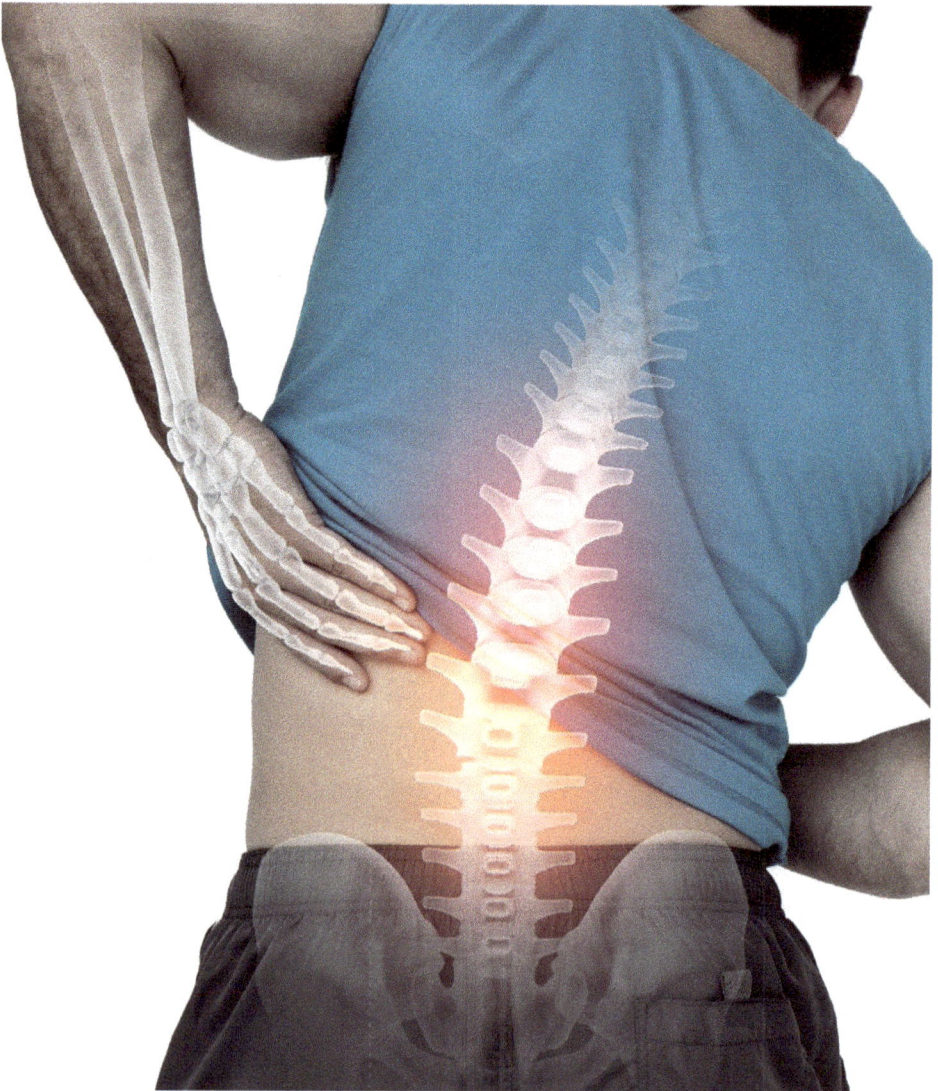

IS IT BETTER TO REST OR STAY ACTIVE WHEN MANAGING BACK PAIN?

When managing back pain, it is better to stay active rather than rest completely, although the approach can vary depending on the severity and type of pain you're experiencing. Here's a detailed look at why staying active is typically recommended, along with guidance on when rest might be necessary:

Staying Active: Benefits and Guidelines

Benefits of Staying Active

Prevents Muscle Weakness and Stiffness

Prolonged rest can lead to muscle atrophy (weakening) and joint stiffness, which can exacerbate back pain and make it more difficult to recover.

Promotes Blood Flow and Healing

Physical activity increases blood circulation, which helps deliver essential nutrients and oxygen to the tissues, promoting healing.

Supports Flexibility and Mobility

Regular movement helps maintain flexibility and mobility in the spine and surrounding muscles, which is crucial for reducing pain and preventing further injury.

Improves Mood and Reduces Stress

Physical activity releases endorphins, which are natural pain relievers and mood enhancers. Staying active can help alleviate stress and anxiety, which are often linked to chronic pain.

Prevents Chronic Pain

Staying active can prevent acute back pain from becoming chronic by keeping the muscles and joints engaged and reducing the risk of developing compensatory movement patterns.

Guidelines for Staying Active

Engage in Low-Impact Activities

- **Walking:** Gentle on the back and helps maintain mobility without putting too much strain on the spine.

- **Swimming or Water Therapy:** The buoyancy of water supports your body and reduces stress on your back while allowing for a full range of motion.

- **Cycling (Stationary Bike):** Provides a low-impact cardiovascular workout that is easier on the back than high-impact activities like running.

Incorporate Gentle Stretching and Strengthening Exercises

- Focus on exercises that strengthen the core muscles and improve flexibility, such as pelvic tilts, bridges, and gentle yoga or pilates.

Listen to Your Body

- While staying active is beneficial, it's important to avoid activities that cause sharp or intense pain. Modify or avoid movements that exacerbate your symptoms.

Maintain Good Posture

- Whether sitting, standing, or exercising, be mindful of your posture to reduce strain on your back. Use ergonomic supports if necessary.

Gradually Increase Activity

- Start with short, gentle activities and gradually increase the intensity and duration as your pain improves and your strength returns.

When Rest is Necessary

When to Consider Resting

Severe Acute Pain

If your back pain is severe or the result of a recent injury (such as a fall or lifting something heavy), a short period of rest may be necessary to allow the initial inflammation and pain to subside.

Pain with Specific Movements

If certain activities or movements consistently worsen your pain, it might be wise to temporarily avoid them until your condition improves.

Neurological Symptoms

If your back pain is accompanied by symptoms such as numbness, tingling, or weakness in the legs, or if you experience loss of bladder or bowel control, you should rest and seek immediate medical attention, as these may indicate a serious condition like a herniated disc or spinal stenosis.

Guidelines for Resting

Short-Term Rest

- If rest is necessary, limit it to short periods (1-2 days) to avoid the negative effects of prolonged inactivity. Resting in a comfortable position, such as lying on your back with a pillow under your knees, can help relieve pain.

Active Rest

- Even during rest periods, try to perform gentle movements such as stretching, light walking, or changing positions frequently to prevent stiffness.

Gradual Return to Activity:

- After a brief period of rest, gradually resume light activities to re-engage your muscles and support the healing process.

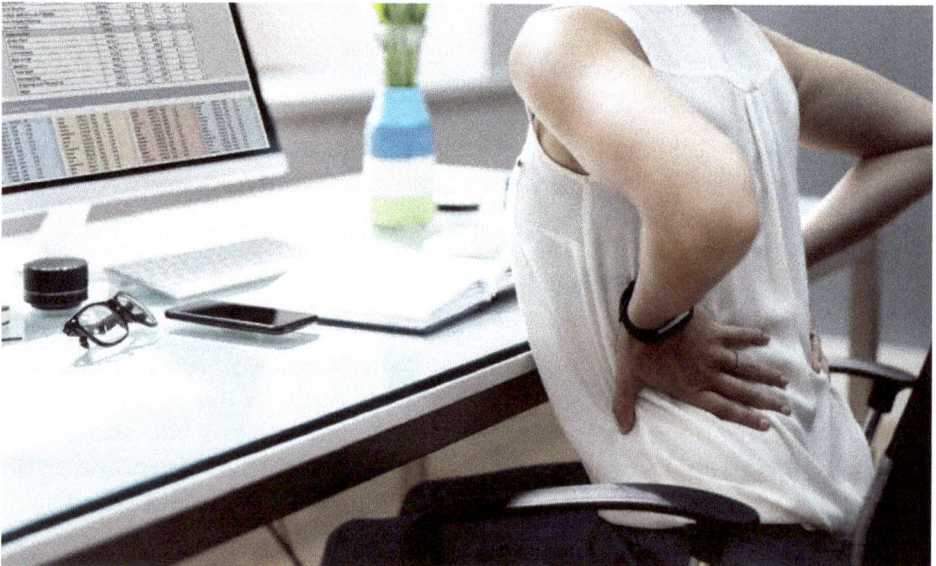

Generally

- In most cases, staying active is better for managing back pain than prolonged rest. Gentle, low-impact activities, combined with proper posture and body mechanics, can help reduce pain, improve mobility, and prevent future episodes of back pain. However, if your pain is severe or associated with other concerning symptoms, a short period of rest may be necessary, followed by a gradual return to activity.

-

- Always listen to your body and consult a healthcare provider if you're unsure about how much activity is safe for your specific condition. They can provide specific advice and guide you on the best approach to managing your back pain.

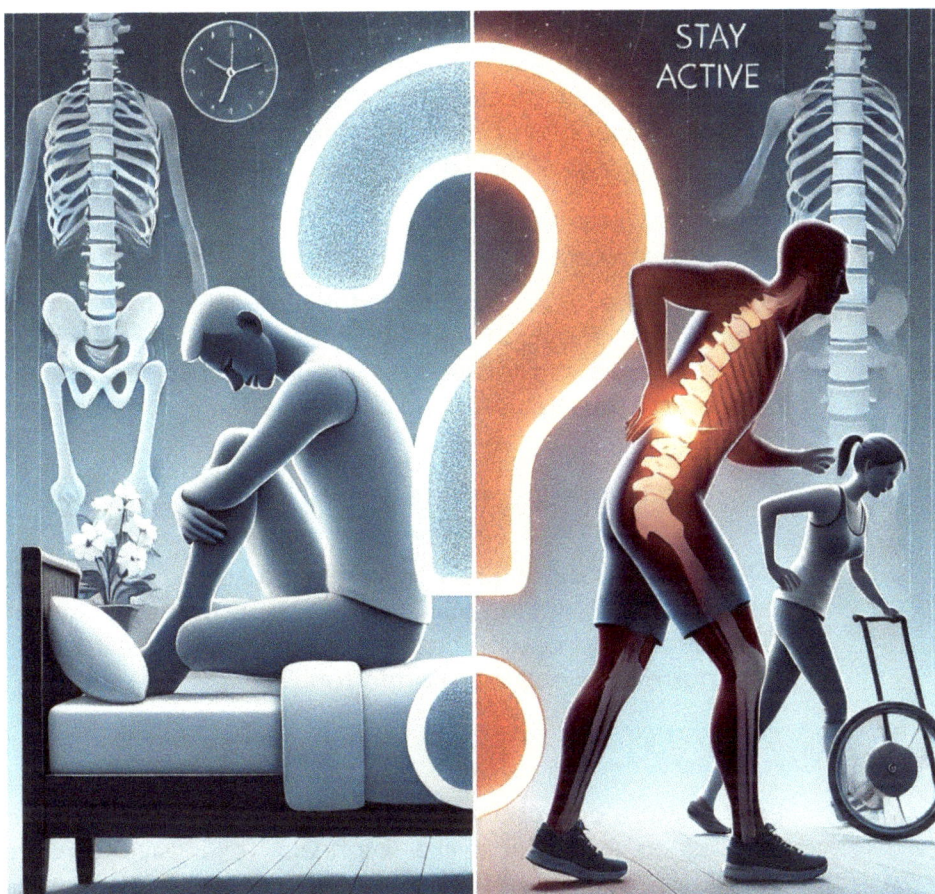

WHAT ROLE DOES POSTURE PLAY IN MANAGING BACK PAIN, AND HOW CAN I IMPROVE MINE?

Posture plays a crucial role in managing and preventing back pain. Proper posture ensures that your spine is aligned correctly, reducing unnecessary stress on the muscles, ligaments, and discs that support your back. On the other hand, poor posture can lead to muscle imbalances, increased strain on the spine, and eventually, back pain. Here's a closer look at how posture affects back pain and strategies for improving your posture:

Impact of Poor Posture on Back Pain

Increased Spinal Stress

Poor posture, such as slouching or hunching over, places uneven loads or pressure on the spine. This can lead to increased wear and tear on the vertebrae and discs, contributing to pain and discomfort.

Muscle Imbalances

Poor posture can cause certain muscles to become overworked and tight, while others become weak. For example, slouching can lead to tight chest muscles and weak upper back muscles, creating an imbalance that contributes to back pain.

Decreased Flexibility and Mobility

Over time, poor posture can cause muscles and joints to become stiff, reducing your flexibility and range of motion. This stiffness can exacerbate back pain and make it harder to perform daily activities comfortably.

Altered Spinal Alignment

Poor posture can change the natural curves of your spine, leading to conditions like kyphosis (excessive forward curvature of the upper spine) or lordosis (excessive inward curvature of the lower spine), both of which can cause pain.

How Good Posture Helps Manage Back Pain

Even Distribution of Pressure

Good posture ensures that the pressure on your spine is evenly distributed, reducing the risk of strain and injury to the vertebrae and discs.

Balanced Muscle Use

Maintaining proper posture engages the core and back muscles in a balanced way, helping to strengthen the muscles that support your spine and reduce the likelihood of pain.

Improved Flexibility and Mobility

Good posture helps maintain the natural alignment of your spine, allowing for better flexibility and mobility. This reduces the risk of stiffness and pain, particularly in the lower back.

Prevention of Future Injuries

By maintaining good posture, you reduce the risk of developing muscle imbalances, disc problems, and other conditions that can lead to chronic back pain.

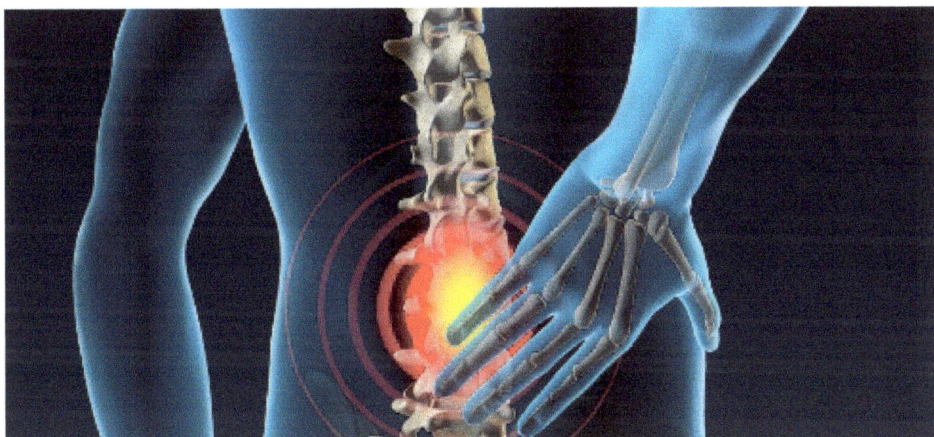

Tips for Improving Your Posture

Sitting Posture

Sit Upright

Sit with your back straight, shoulders relaxed, and your buttocks touching the back of the chair. Avoid slouching or leaning forward.

Use Lumbar Support

Place a small pillow or lumbar roll behind your lower back to maintain the natural curve of your spine. This helps reduce strain on the lower back.

Feet Flat on the Floor

Keep your feet flat on the floor or on a footrest, with your knees bent at a 90-degree angle and slightly higher than your hips.

Adjust Your Chair

Ensure that your chair is adjusted so that your thighs are parallel to the ground and your arms are at a 90-degree angle when typing or using a mouse.

Position Your Screen

Place your computer monitor at eye level, about an arm's length away, to avoid straining your neck and upper back.

Standing Posture

Align Your Ears, Shoulders, and Hips

Stand with your ears, shoulders, and hips in a straight line. Avoid leaning forward or arching your lower back excessively.

Distribute Your Weight Evenly

Keep your weight evenly distributed on both feet. Avoid leaning on one leg or shifting your weight to one side for extended periods.

Engage Your Core

Slightly engage your abdominal muscles to support your lower back and maintain the natural curve of your spine.

Use a Footrest

If you need to stand for long periods, place one foot on a small stool or footrest to relieve pressure on your lower back. Alternate feet periodically.

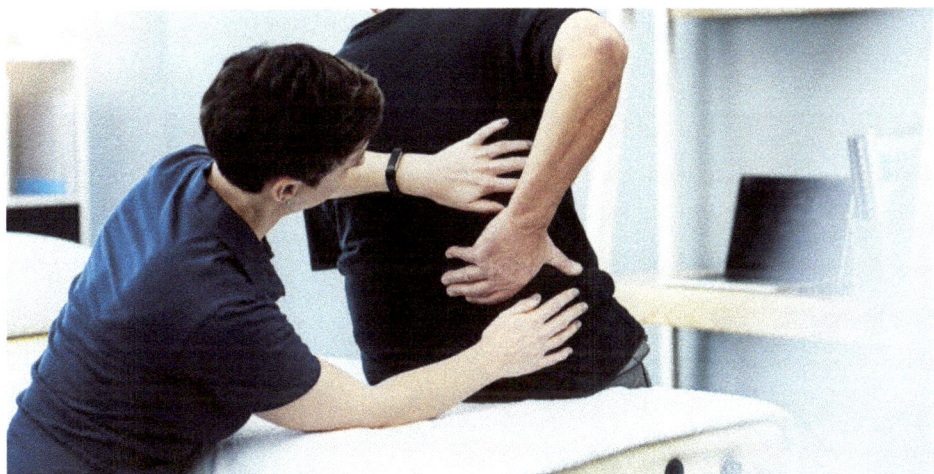

Sleeping Posture

Use a Supportive Mattress

Choose a mattress that provides adequate support for your spine and maintains its natural alignment. Avoid overly soft or sagging mattresses.

Sleep on Your Back or Side

Sleeping on your back with a pillow under your knees or on your side with a pillow between your knees helps maintain the natural curve of your spine.

Avoid Stomach Sleeping

Sleeping on your stomach can strain your neck and back, leading to pain. If possible, switch to a back or side sleeping position.

Use the Right Pillow

Use a pillow that supports your neck and keeps your head in alignment with your spine. For side sleepers, a thicker pillow may be needed to fill the space between your neck and the mattress.

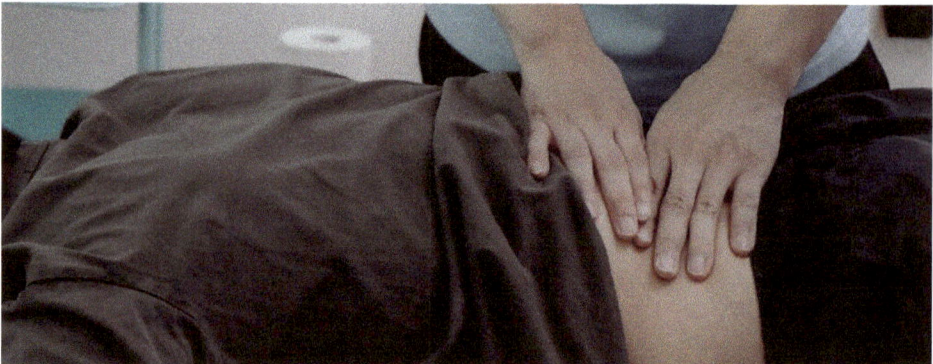

Lifting and Carrying Posture

Bend at Your Knees

When lifting objects, bend at your knees and hips rather than your waist. Keep your back straight and lift with your leg muscles.

Hold Objects Close to Your Body

Keep the object close to your body at waist level to reduce the strain on your back.

Avoid Twisting

Avoid twisting your body while lifting or carrying objects. Instead, turn your whole body by moving your feet.

Use Assistive Devices

If you need to stand for long periods, place one foot on a small stool or footrest to relieve pressure on your lower back. Alternate feet periodically.

Summarising all the above it is recommended that good posture is essential for managing and preventing back pain. By making conscious efforts to maintain proper posture throughout your daily activities—whether sitting, standing, sleeping, or lifting—you can reduce the strain on your spine, improve your overall spinal health, and decrease the likelihood of experiencing back pain.

Improving your posture may take time and practice, but the benefits for your back and overall well-being are significant. If you're unsure about your posture or need additional guidance, consider consulting a physical therapist or healthcare provider for personalised advice and exercises to help you achieve and maintain good posture.

HOW CAN I MANAGE BACK PAIN FLARE-UPS WHEN THEY OCCUR?

Managing back pain flare-ups effectively involves a combination of immediate relief strategies, ongoing self-care, and preventive measures to reduce the severity and duration of the pain. Here's a comprehensive guide to help you manage back pain flare-ups when they occur:

Immediate Relief Strategies

Rest (Short-Term)

• **What to Do:**
  Take a break from activities that may have triggered the flare-up. Rest in a comfortable position that supports your back, such as lying on your back with a pillow under your knees or lying on your side with a pillow between your knees.

• **Why It Helps:**
  Resting briefly allows your muscles and spine to relax, reducing the stress on the affected area. However, avoid prolonged bed rest, as it can lead to stiffness and muscle weakness.

Cold Therapy

• **What to Do:**
  Apply an ice pack or cold compress to the painful area for 15-20 minutes, several times a day, especially within the first 48 hours of the flare-up.

• **Why It Helps:**
  Cold therapy helps reduce inflammation, numb the area, and alleviate pain by constricting blood vessels and reducing swelling.

Heat Therapy

- **What to Do:**
  After the initial 48 hours or if the pain is due to muscle tension or spasms, switch to heat therapy. Apply a heating pad, warm compress, or take a warm bath for 15-20 minutes.

- **Why It Helps:**
  Heat therapy increases blood flow to the affected area, relaxes tight muscles, and helps alleviate pain and stiffness.

Over the Counter Pain Relief (speak to your doctor)

- **What to Do:**
  Take over the counter pain relief like paracetamol or nonsteroidal anti-inflammatory drugs (NSAIDs) as directed.

- **Why It Helps:**
  These medications can help reduce pain and inflammation, providing temporary relief during a flare-up.

Gentle Stretching

- **What to Do:**
  Perform gentle stretches that target the back, hips, and hamstrings. Avoid aggressive or intense stretching during a flare-up.

- **Why It Helps:**
  Stretching helps maintain flexibility, reduces muscle tension, and prevents stiffness, which can worsen back pain.

Mind-Body Techniques

- **What to Do:**
  Practice relaxation techniques such as deep breathing, mindfulness meditation, or progressive muscle relaxation to manage stress and reduce pain perception.

- **Why It Helps:**
  Stress can exacerbate pain, so managing it through relaxation techniques can help you cope better during a flare-up.

Ongoing Self-Care

Gradual Return to Activity

- **What to Do:**
  As your pain begins to subside, gradually resume normal activities. Start with low-impact exercises like walking or swimming and avoid high-intensity activities until your back has fully recovered.

- **Why It Helps:**
  Gradually resuming activity helps prevent muscle stiffness and weakness and supports overall recovery.

Maintain Good Posture

- **What to Do:**
  Pay attention to your posture while sitting, standing, and lifting. Use ergonomic supports and adjust your workspace if needed.

- **Why It Helps:**
  Proper posture reduces strain on your spine and helps prevent future flare-ups.

Continue with Core Strengthening Exercises

- **What to Do:**
  Incorporate exercises that strengthen your core muscles into your routine, such as planks, bridges, and pelvic tilts.

- **Why It Helps:**
  A strong core provides better support for your spine and helps reduce the risk of future back pain episodes.

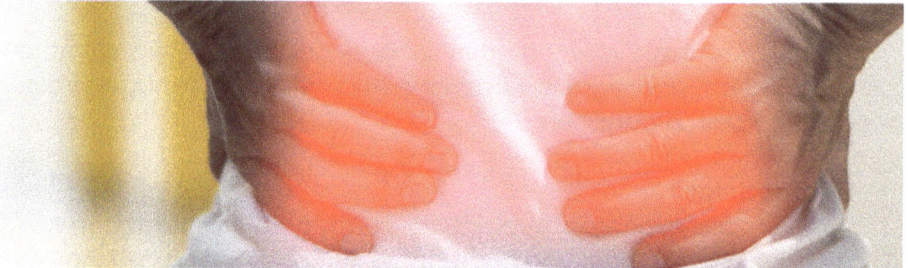

Use Supportive Footwear

- **What to Do:**
  Wear shoes with good arch support and cushioning, especially if you spend long hours on your feet. Consider orthotic inserts if necessary.

- **Why It Helps:**
  Proper footwear helps maintain good posture and reduces the strain on your back during daily activities.

Preventive Measures

Regular Exercise

- **What to Do:**
  Engage in regular physical activity, including low-impact aerobic exercises, strength training, and flexibility exercises.

- **Why It Helps:**
  Regular exercise helps maintain a healthy weight, strengthens the muscles that support your back, and improves flexibility, all of which reduce the risk of future flare-ups.

Weight Management

- **What to Do:**
  Maintain a healthy weight through a balanced diet and regular exercise. If you are overweight, consider a weight loss plan to reduce the strain on your back.

- **Why It Helps:**
  Excess weight, particularly around the abdomen, puts additional pressure on the spine and can contribute to back pain.

Ergonomics at Work and Home

- **What to Do:**
  Ensure that your workstation is ergonomically designed to support good posture and reduce strain. Use a chair with lumbar support,

position your computer screen at eye level, and take regular breaks to move and stretch.

- **Why It Helps:**
  Proper ergonomics reduce the risk of developing back pain from prolonged sitting, standing, or repetitive tasks.

Mind-Body Practices

- **What to Do:**
  Incorporate stress-reduction techniques into your daily routine, such as yoga, tai chi, or meditation.

- **Why It Helps:**
  Managing stress effectively can prevent muscle tension and reduce the likelihood of back pain flare-ups.

Avoid Heavy Lifting

- **What to Do:**
  Use proper lifting techniques, bend at your knees, keep the object close to your body, and lift with your legs, not your back. Avoid lifting heavy objects if possible and seek help when needed.

- **Why It Helps:**
  Proper lifting techniques prevent strain and reduce the risk of injury to your back.

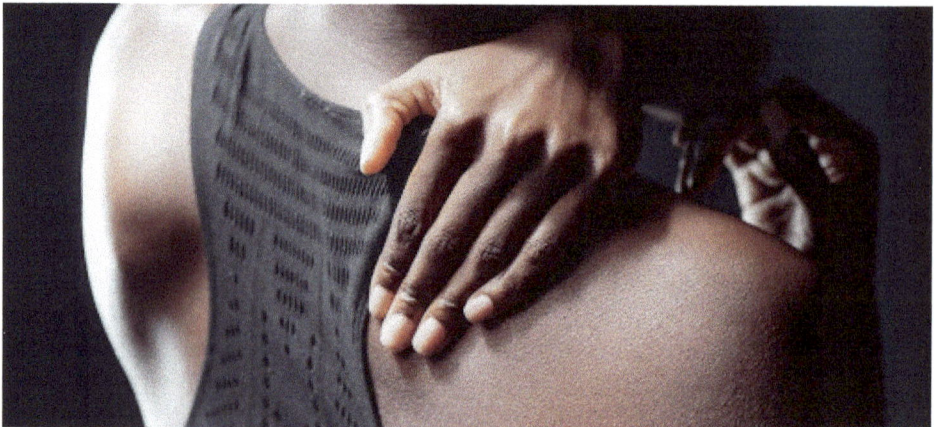

When to Seek Medical Help

Persistent or Worsening Pain

- If your back pain does not improve after a few days of self-care or if it worsens, seek medical attention to rule out any underlying conditions.

Neurological Symptoms

- If you experience numbness, tingling, weakness, or loss of bladder or bowel control, seek immediate medical attention, as these could indicate a serious condition like a herniated disc or spinal stenosis.

Frequent Flare-Ups

- If you experience frequent back pain flare-ups, consult a healthcare provider or physical therapist for a comprehensive evaluation and treatment plan.

Managing back pain flare-ups involves a combination of immediate relief strategies, ongoing self-care, and preventive measures. By staying proactive and addressing flare-ups promptly, you can reduce their severity and duration, minimise discomfort, and prevent future occurrences. If your pain persists or worsens, or if you have any concerns, it's important to consult a healthcare provider for further evaluation and guidance.

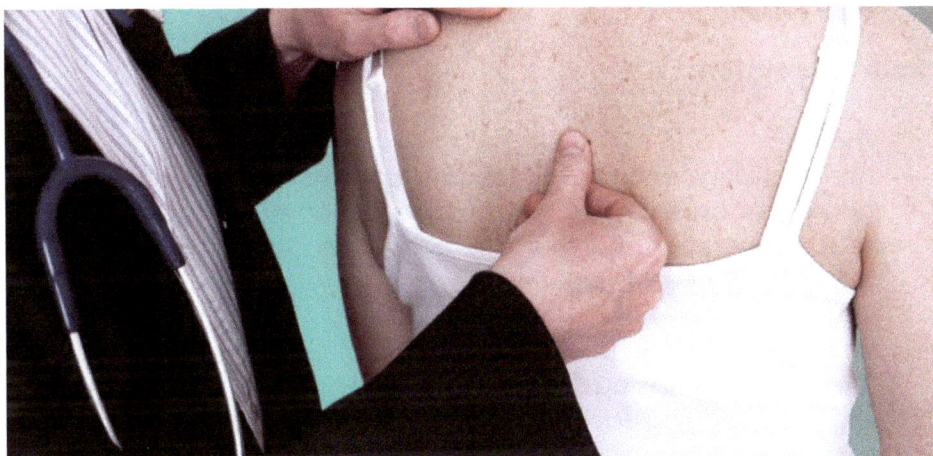

WHAT ROLES DO STRESS AND MENTAL HEALTH PLAY IN MANAGING BACK PAIN, AND HOW CAN I ADDRESS THEM?

Stress and mental health are closely linked to the experience and management of back pain. While back pain is often associated with physical factors, psychological aspects such as stress, anxiety, and depression can significantly influence both the perception of pain and the effectiveness of treatment. Understanding the role of these factors and addressing them as part of a comprehensive pain management plan can lead to better outcomes.

How Stress and Mental Health Affect Back Pain

Increased Muscle Tension:

*   **Impact:**
    When you are stressed or anxious, your body may respond with increased muscle tension, particularly in the neck, shoulders, and back. This tension can lead to muscle stiffness, spasms, and pain, exacerbating existing back issues.

*   **Mechanism:**
    Stress triggers the body's "fight or flight" response, releasing stress hormones like cortisol and adrenaline. These hormones can cause muscles to tighten, particularly around areas of the body that are already vulnerable.

Pain Perception:

*   **Impact:**
    Stress, anxiety, and depression can amplify the perception of pain. Individuals experiencing elevated levels of stress or poor mental health may report more intense pain, even if the physical condition of their back hasn't worsened.

*   **Mechanism:**
    The brain's processing of pain signals can be influenced by emotional and psychological factors. Stress and negative emotions can lower pain thresholds, making individuals more sensitive to pain.

Sleep Disruption:

- **Impact:**
  Stress and anxiety can interfere with sleep, leading to poor quality or insufficient rest. Lack of sleep can worsen back pain by reducing the body's ability to heal and recover from daily strain.

- **Mechanism:**
  During sleep, the body repairs tissues and reduces inflammation. Chronic stress and poor mental health can disrupt sleep patterns, leading to a vicious cycle of pain and sleep deprivation.

Behavioural Impact:

- **Impact:**
  Individuals under stress or experiencing depression may engage in behaviour that worsen back pain, such as inactivity, poor posture, or substance use (e.g., smoking, alcohol).

- **Mechanism:**
  Stress can lead to coping mechanisms that are detrimental to physical health, such as avoiding exercise or neglecting self-care routines. Additionally, stress-related behaviour can contribute to weight gain, which adds further strain on the back.

Treatment Adherence:

- **Impact:**
  Mental health challenges can affect an individual's ability to adhere to treatment plans, including exercise regimens, physical therapy, and medication schedules.

- **Mechanism:**
  Depression and anxiety can reduce motivation and energy levels, making it difficult to follow through with prescribed treatments, leading to poorer outcomes.

Addressing Stress and Mental Health to Manage Back Pain

Mindfulness and Relaxation Techniques

- **What to Do:**
  When you are stressed or anxious, your body may respond with increased muscle tension, particularly in the neck, shoulders, and back. This tension can lead to muscle stiffness, spasms, and pain, exacerbating existing back issues.

- **How It Helps:**
  These techniques help calm the nervous system, reduce muscle tension, and improve pain perception by encouraging a focus on the present moment rather than on pain or stressors.

Cognitive-Behavioural Therapy (CBT)

- **What to Do:**
  Consider working with a therapist trained in CBT, a form of therapy that helps individuals identify and change negative thought patterns and behaviour related to pain and stress.

- **How It Helps:**
  CBT can help reduce the psychological impact of pain, improve coping strategies, and decrease the intensity of pain by addressing the way you think about and respond to pain.

Exercise and Physical Activity

- **What to Do:**
  Engage in regular physical activity, such as walking, swimming, or yoga, which can help reduce stress and improve mood.

- **How It Helps:**
  Exercise releases endorphins, the body's natural painkillers, and mood elevators. Physical activity also helps reduce muscle tension and improves sleep quality, both of which are beneficial for managing back pain.

Sleep Hygiene

- **What to Do:**
  Establish a regular sleep routine by going to bed and waking up at the same time each day, creating a relaxing bedtime routine, and ensuring your sleep environment is conducive to rest.

- **How It Helps:**
  Good sleep hygiene improves sleep quality, which is essential for pain management and overall mental health. Addressing sleep issues can also help break the cycle of pain and poor sleep.

Social Support

- **What to Do:**
  Reach out to friends, family, or support groups for emotional support and encouragement.

- **How It Helps:**
  Social connections can help reduce feelings of isolation, provide comfort, and improve your ability to cope with stress and pain. Talking about your experiences can also lead to valuable advice and insights from others who have faced similar challenges.

Healthy Lifestyle Choices

- **What to Do:**
  Maintain a balanced diet, avoid excessive alcohol consumption, and quit smoking, as these habits can negatively affect both physical and mental health.

- **How It Helps:**
  A healthy lifestyle supports overall well-being, reduces inflammation, and improves the body's ability to manage stress and pain. Avoiding smoking and excessive alcohol use is particularly important, as these can exacerbate both pain and mental health issues.

Medication Management

- **What to Do:**
  If stress or mental health issues are significantly impacting your life and pain management, consult a healthcare provider about the possibility of using medications such as antidepressants or anti-anxiety medications.

- **How It Helps:**
  Medications can help manage symptoms of depression or anxiety, improving your overall mood and reducing the impact of stress on your back pain. Antidepressants can also sometimes help with chronic pain by affecting neurotransmitters in the brain that influence pain perception.

Time Management and Prioritisationt

- **What to Do:**
  Manage your time effectively by setting realistic goals, prioritising tasks, and taking breaks when needed. Avoid overcommitting and learn to say no when necessary.

- **How It Helps:**
  Reducing the burden of daily stressors and avoiding unnecessary stress can help prevent exacerbation of back pain. Time management also allows you to dedicate time to self-care and relaxation, which are crucial for managing both stress and pain.

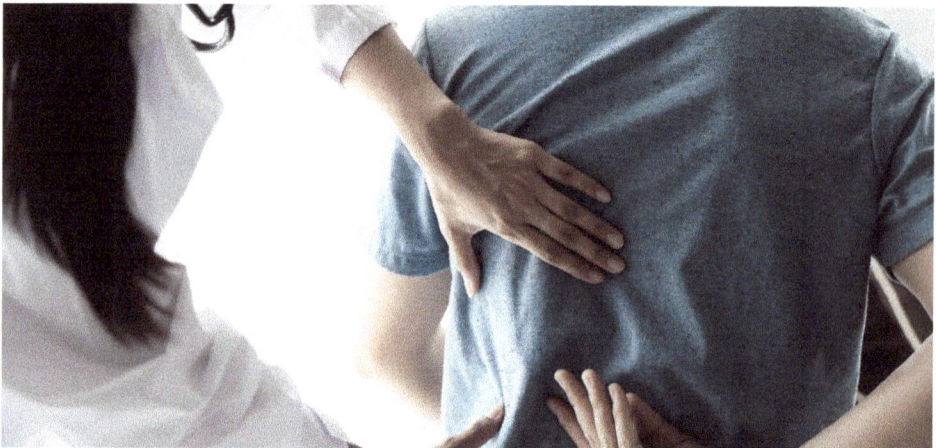

Conclusion

Stress and mental health play a significant role in managing back pain, influencing everything from pain perception to treatment adherence. By addressing these psychological factors through relaxation techniques, therapy, exercise, and lifestyle changes, you can improve your ability to manage back pain effectively. A holistic approach that considers both physical and mental well-being is essential for long-term pain management and overall quality of life.

If you find that stress or mental health challenges are significantly affecting your ability to manage back pain, it's important to seek help from a healthcare provider or mental health professional who can provide personalised support and guidance.

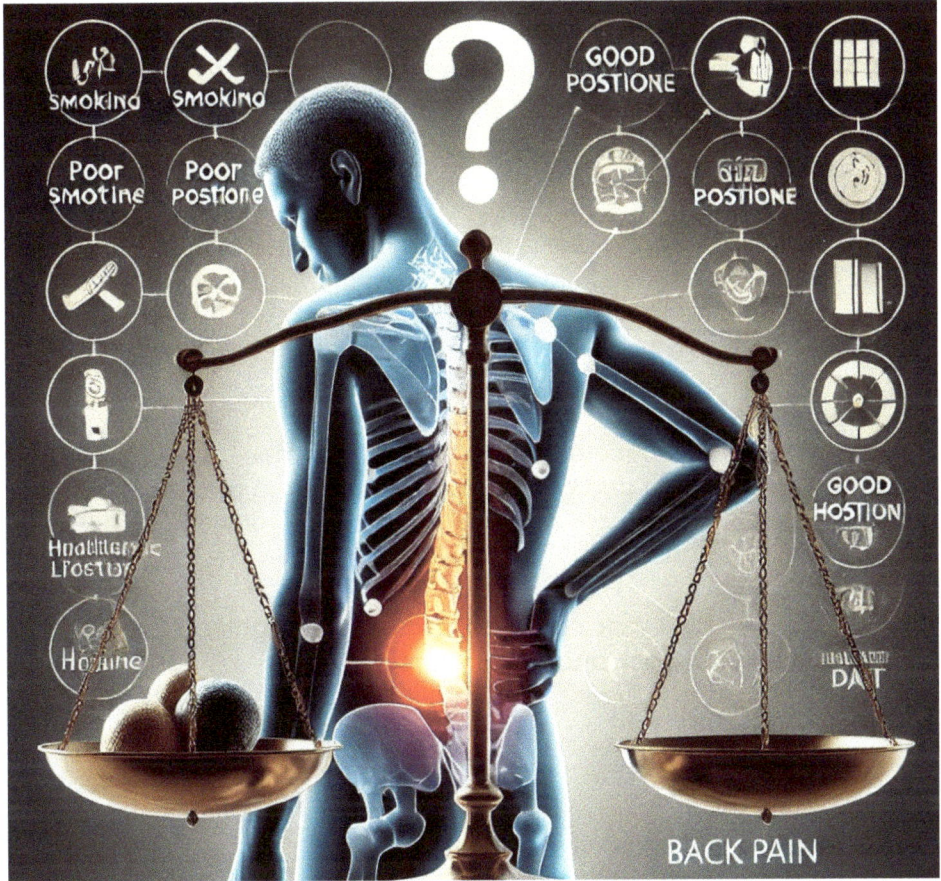

CAN DIET AND NUTRITION IMPACT MY BACK PAIN, AND WHAT FOODS SHOULD I EAT OR AVOID?

Diet and nutrition can have a significant impact on back pain. The foods you eat can influence inflammation levels in your body, contribute to your overall weight, and affect bone and muscle health, all of which play a role in managing or exacerbating back pain. By making mindful dietary choices, you can support your back health and potentially reduce pain. Here's how diet and nutrition impact back pain and which foods to include or avoid:

How Diet and Nutrition Impact Back Pain

Inflammation

- **Impact:**
  Chronic inflammation in the body can contribute to pain, including back pain. Certain foods can either promote or reduce inflammation, affecting how you feel.

- **Role of Diet:**
  An anti-inflammatory diet can help manage chronic pain conditions by reducing systemic inflammation.

Weight Management

- **Impact:**
  Excess weight, particularly around the abdomen, places additional stress on the spine and back muscles, increasing the risk of pain and injury.

- **Role of Diet:**
  A balanced diet that supports a healthy weight can reduce the burden on your back and lower your risk of pain.

Bone Health

- **Impact:**
  The health of your bones, including the vertebrae in your spine, is directly related to your nutrient intake, particularly calcium and vitamin D. Poor bone health can lead to conditions like osteoporosis, which increases the risk of fractures and back pain.

- **Role of Diet:**
  A diet rich in bone-supporting nutrients helps maintain strong bones and reduces the risk of spine-related issues.

Muscle Function

- **Impact:**
  Strong and healthy muscles support the spine and help prevent back pain. Nutrients like protein, magnesium, and potassium are essential for muscle function and recovery.

- **Role of Diet:**
  Consuming adequate amounts of these nutrients supports muscle health and reduces the risk of muscle-related back pain.

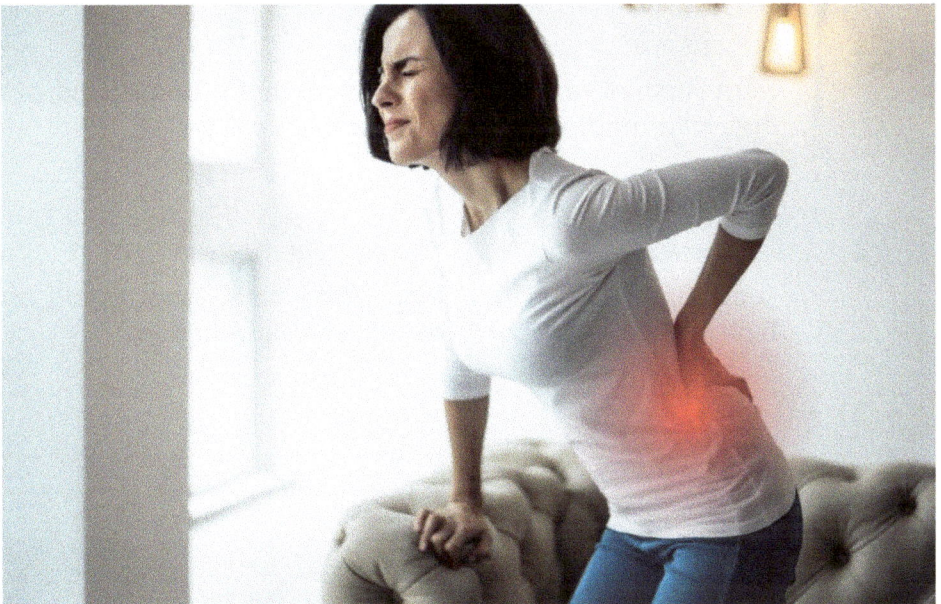

Foods to Eat for Better Back Health

Anti-Inflammatory Foods:

Fatty Fish

Salmon, mackerel, and sardines are rich in omega-3 fatty acids, which have powerful anti-inflammatory properties.

Fruits and Vegetables

Berries, leafy greens, tomatoes, and other colourful fruits and vegetables are high in antioxidants that help reduce inflammation.

Nuts and Seeds:

Walnuts, chia seeds are good sources of omega-3s and anti-inflammatory compounds.

Olive Oil

Extra virgin olive oil contains oleocanthal, a compound with anti-inflammatory effects similar to ibuprofen.

Whole Grains

Foods like brown rice, quinoa, and whole wheat bread are high in fibre, which can help reduce inflammation.

Bone-Strengthening Foods:

Dairy Products

Milk, yogurt, and cheese are rich in calcium and often fortified with vitamin D, which are essential for bone health.

Leafy Greens

Kale, broccoli, and spinach provide calcium, magnesium, and vitamin K, all of which are important for bone health.

Fortified Foods

Some plant-based milks, orange juice, and cereals are fortified with calcium and vitamin D.

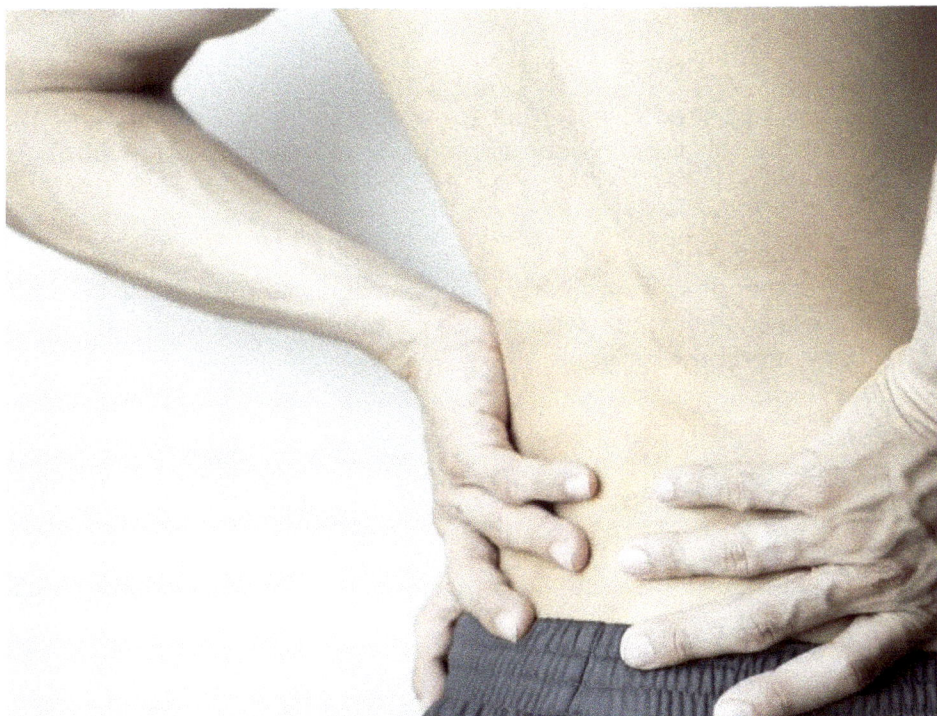

Muscle-Supporting Foods

Lean Protein

Chicken, turkey, tofu, and legumes provide the protein needed for muscle repair and strength.

Magnesium-Rich Foods

Spinach, almonds, and avocados are high in magnesium, which supports muscle function and relaxation.

Potassium-Rich Foods

Bananas, sweet potatoes, and beans help maintain muscle function and prevent cramps.

Hydration

*   **Water:**
    Staying hydrated is essential for maintaining the elasticity of the intervertebral discs in your spine. Drink plenty of water throughout the day.

*   **Herbal Teas:**
    Non-caffeinated herbal teas can be a suitable alternative to water and provide hydration without the potential inflammatory effects of caffeinated beverages.

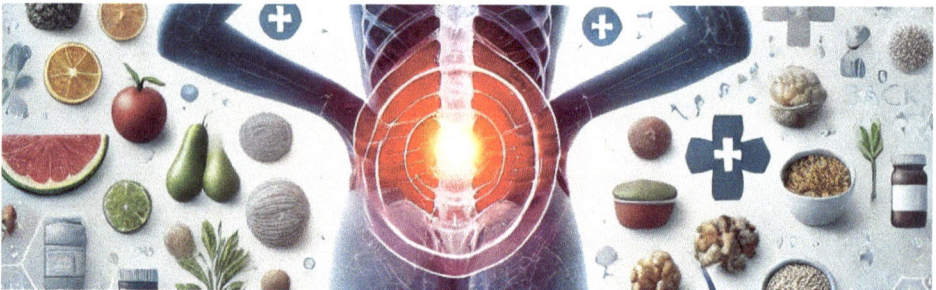

Foods to Avoid or Limit

Processed Foods

- **Why to Avoid:**
  Processed foods like chips, cookies, and fast food are often high in trans fats, sugars, and refined carbohydrates, which can promote inflammation.

- **Impact on Back Pain:**
  These foods can increase systemic inflammation, potentially worsening back pain.

Energy Drinks, Sodas, and Snacks

- **Why to Avoid:**
  These drinks and snacks cause spikes in blood sugar levels and promote inflammation.

- **Impact on Back Pain:**
  High sugar intake is associated with increased inflammation, which can exacerbate pain.

Refined Grains

- **Why to Avoid:**
  White bread, white rice, and other refined grains are stripped of their nutrients and can contribute to inflammation.

- **Impact on Back Pain:**
  Refined grains can promote weight gain and inflammation, both of which can aggravate back pain.

High-Sodium Foods

- **Why to Avoid:**
  Processed and packaged foods are often high in sodium, which can lead to water retention and increased blood pressure.

- **Impact on Back Pain:**
  High sodium intake can contribute to swelling and discomfort, including in the back.

Alcohol

- **Why to Avoid:**
  Alcohol can dehydrate the body, leading to disc degeneration and increased back pain. It can also interfere with sleep, which is crucial for recovery.

- **Impact on Back Pain:**
  Excessive alcohol consumption can exacerbate inflammation and negatively affect sleep and recovery, worsening back pain.

Caffeine

- **Why to Avoid:**
  While moderate caffeine intake is safe, excessive consumption can contribute to dehydration and disrupt sleep.

- **Impact on Back Pain:**
  Dehydration and poor sleep can both contribute to back pain

In conclusion, diet and nutrition play a significant role in managing back pain. By focusing on anti-inflammatory foods, maintaining a healthy weight, and ensuring you get enough nutrients to support bone and muscle health, you can reduce the risk of back pain and improve your overall well-being. Conversely, limiting processed foods, sugars, refined grains, and other inflammatory foods can help prevent exacerbation of pain. If you're unsure about the best dietary approach for managing your back pain, consider consulting with a healthcare provider or a registered dietitian who can provide personalised guidance based on your individual needs and health conditions.

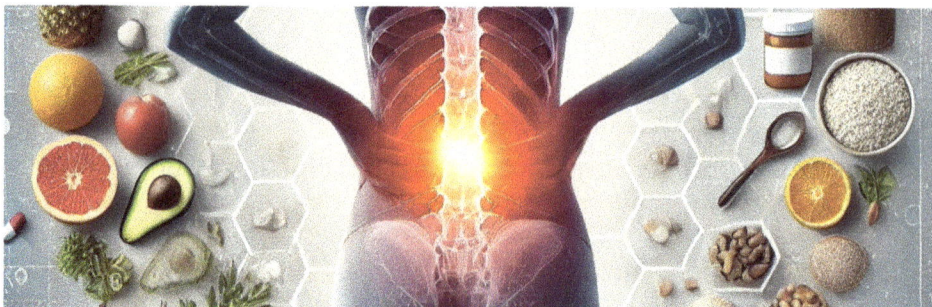

GENERAL QUESTIONS ABOUT ERGONOMICS IN BACK PAIN

These questions focus on how to optimise one's environment and habits to reduce back strain and prevent back pain, particularly in settings like the workplace or home office.

WHAT IS THE BEST TYPE OF CHAIR TO USE AT WORK TO PREVENT OR MANAGE BACK PAIN?

Choosing the right chair for work is crucial in preventing or managing back pain, especially if you spend long hours sitting. An ergonomic chair is considered the best type for supporting your back and promoting good posture. Here are the key features to look for in a chair to help prevent or manage back pain:

Key Features of an Ergonomic Chair

Lumbar Support

- **Why It Matters:**
  Processed foods like chips, cookies, and fast food are often high in trans fats, sugars, and refined carbohydrates, which can promote inflammation.

- **What to Look For:**
  - A chair with adjustable lumbar support that can be positioned to match the curve of your lower back.

  - Some chairs offer a built-in lumbar support cushion, while others allow you to adjust the depth and height of the support.

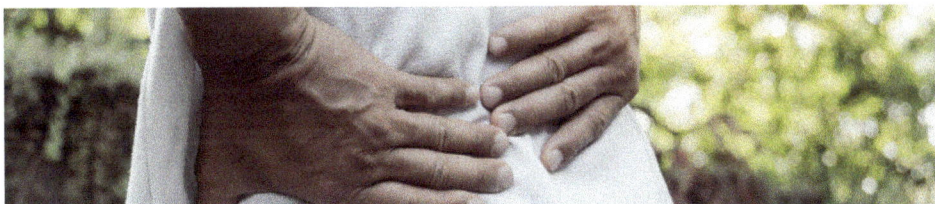

Adjustable Seat Height

- **Why It Matters:**
  Adjusting the seat height ensures that your feet are flat on the floor and your knees are at a 90-degree angle, which helps distribute your body weight evenly and reduces strain on your lower back.

- **What to Look For:**
  - A chair with a pneumatic adjustment lever that allows you to easily change the seat height.

  - Ensure the seat height can be adjusted so that your thighs are parallel to the floor.

Seat Depth and Width

- **Why It Matters:**
  Proper seat depth ensures that you have enough support under your thighs without putting pressure on the back of your knees. This helps promote circulation and reduces lower back strain.

- **What to Look For:**
  - A seat depth that allows you to sit back comfortably against the lumbar support with 2-4 inches (5-10 centimetres) of space between the back of your knees and the front edge of the seat.

  - A seat width that comfortably supports your hips without being too narrow or too wide.

Adjustable Backrest

- **Why It Matters:**
  An adjustable backrest allows you to set the angle and height of the backrest to support the natural curve of your spine, reducing the risk of slouching or leaning forward.

- **What to Look For:**
  - A backrest that tilts and locks in place, allowing you to recline slightly while maintaining support for your lower back.

  - A height-adjustable backrest that can be positioned to support your entire back, including the lumbar region.

Seat Cushioning

- **Why It Matters:**
  Proper cushioning provides comfort and support, reducing pressure on your hips and lower back, which can help prevent pain during prolonged sitting.

- **What to Look For:**
  - A chair with high-density foam or memory foam cushioning that provides firm, even support.

  - Avoid overly soft or thin cushioning that may compress over time and fail to provide adequate support.

Armrests

- **Why It Matters:**
  Adjustable armrests help support your arms and shoulders, reducing strain on your upper back and neck. Proper armrest height also helps maintain good posture.

- **What to Look For:**
  - Armrests that are adjustable in height and width to accommodate your specific body size and desk setup.

  - Armrests that allow your arms to rest comfortably at a 90-degree angle, with your shoulders relaxed.

Swivel and Mobility

- **Why It Matters:**
  A chair with a swivel base and smooth-rolling casters allows you to move easily without twisting your spine, reducing the risk of strain.

- **What to Look For:**
  - A chair that swivels 360 degrees to enable easy movement and access to different areas of your workspace.

  - Durable casters that glide smoothly on your floor surface (consider a chair mat if needed to protect your floor).

Recline Function

- **Why It Matters:**
  The ability to recline slightly can help reduce pressure on your lower back and spine by distributing your body weight more evenly.

- **What to Look For:**
  - A chair with a recline function that allows you to tilt the backrest to an angle of 100 to 110 degrees.

  - A recline lock feature to hold the backrest in your preferred position.

Breathable Material

- **Why It Matters:**
  Breathable fabric helps regulate temperature and moisture, keeping you comfortable during long periods of sitting.

- **What to Look For:**
  - A chair with a mesh back that allows for air circulation, or a chair with breathable fabric upholstery.

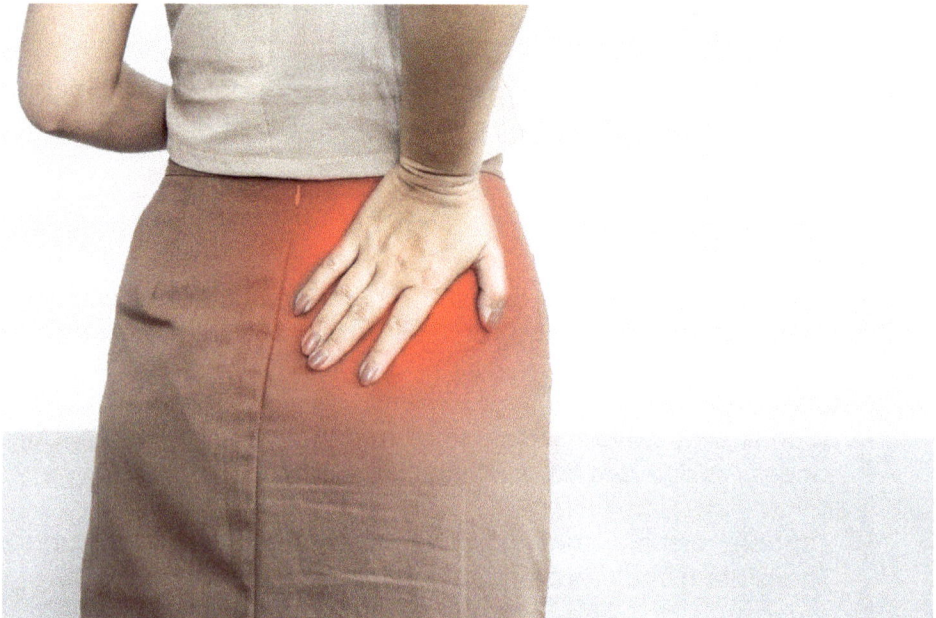

Additional Considerations

Fit for Your Body

Ensure that the chair's dimensions and adjustability suit your body size and shape. A chair that's too large or too small can cause discomfort and exacerbate back pain.

Regular Adjustment

Periodically adjust your chair throughout the day to maintain good posture and prevent stiffness. Change your sitting position, adjust the lumbar support, or recline slightly to relieve pressure on your back.

Use of Accessories

Consider using additional ergonomic accessories, such as a footrest to support your feet if the chair height requires it, or a lumbar roll for extra lower back support.

An ergonomic chair with the right features can significantly reduce the risk of developing or worsening back pain by promoting proper posture and providing adequate support throughout the workday. Investing in a high-quality chair that meets your specific needs can improve your comfort, productivity, and overall spinal health. If possible, try out different chairs to find the one that best supports your back and suits your work environment.

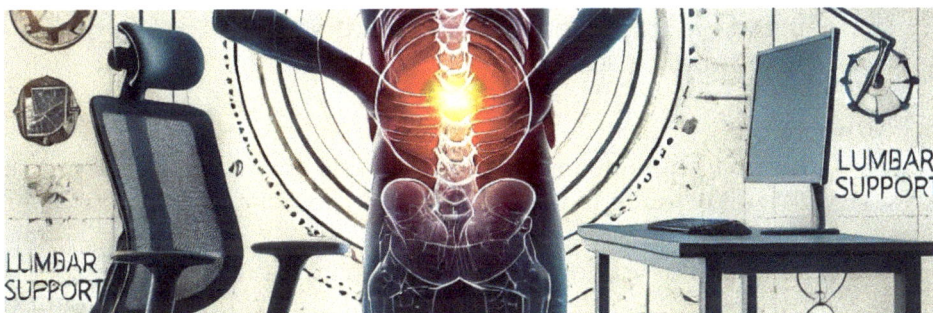

HOW SHOULD MY DESK AND COMPUTER BE SET UP TO MINIMISE BACK STRAIN?

Setting up your desk and computer correctly is essential to minimising back strain and promoting good posture, especially if you spend long hours working at a desk. An ergonomic setup can help reduce the risk of developing back pain and other musculoskeletal issues. Here's how to properly arrange your desk and computer to minimise back strain:

Desk Height and Setup

Correct Desk Height

- **Why It Matters:**
  The height of your desk should allow you to sit comfortably with your feet flat on the floor and your arms at a 90-degree angle while typing. A desk that is too high or too low can lead to poor posture and back strain.

- **What to Do:**
  - Adjust your desk height so that your elbows are at the same height as the keyboard, allowing your arms to form a 90-degree angle when typing.

  - Your desk should provide enough space for your legs to fit comfortably underneath without any restriction.

Desk Surface

- **Why It Matters:**
  Your desk surface should have enough space to accommodate your computer, keyboard, mouse, and any other necessary items while keeping them within easy reach.

- **What to Do:**
  - Arrange frequently used items, such as your mouse and phone, within easy reach to avoid excessive stretching or twisting.

  - Keep your desk organised to reduce clutter and allow for smooth movement.

Chair Position and Posture

Chair Height and Position

- **Why It Matters:**
  Your chair should be adjusted so that your feet are flat on the floor, your knees are at a 90-degree angle, and your hips are slightly higher than your knees.

- **What to Do:**
  - Adjust the height of your chair so that your thighs are parallel to the floor and your feet rest flat on the ground or on a footrest if needed.

  - Sit back in your chair so that your lower back is fully supported by the lumbar support.

Maintain Good Posture

- **Why It Matters:**
  Proper posture reduces strain on your back and spine, helping to prevent pain and discomfort.

- **What to Do:**
  - Sit upright with your shoulders relaxed and your back against the backrest.

  - Keep your ears aligned with your shoulders and avoid leaning forward or slouching.

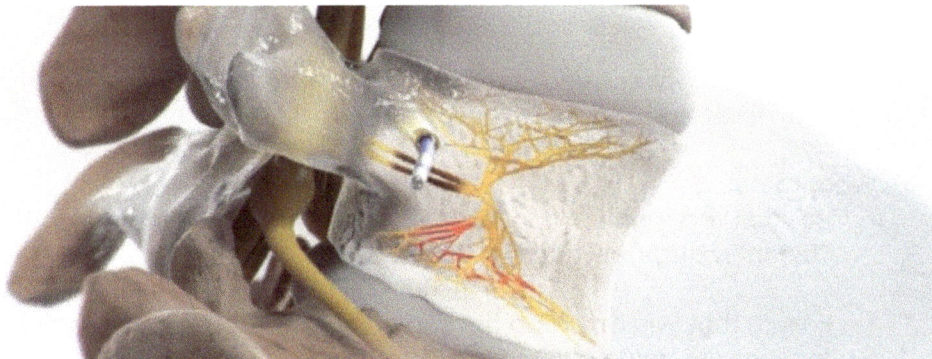

Monitor Placement

Monitor Height

- **Why It Matters:**
  Your computer monitor should be positioned so that the top of the screen is at or slightly below eye level to avoid neck and back strain.

- **What to Do:**
  - Adjust the height of your chair so that your thighs are parallel to the floor and your feet rest flat on the ground or on a footrest if needed.

  - Sit back in your chair so that your lower back is fully supported by the lumbar support.

Maintain Good Posture

- **Why It Matters:**
  Proper posture reduces strain on your back and spine, helping to prevent pain and discomfort.

- **What to Do:**
  - Position the top of the monitor at eye level or slightly below, so you can look straight ahead without tilting your head up or down.

  - If needed, use a monitor stand or stack books under the monitor to raise it to the correct height.

Monitor Distance

- **Why It Matters:**
  The distance between your eyes and the monitor affects your posture and can lead to strain if not set correctly.

- **What to Do:**
  - Position the monitor about an arm's length (20-30 inches or 50-75 centimetres) away from your eyes.

  - Ensure that you can read the screen comfortably without leaning forward or straining your eyes.

Monitor Alignment

- **Why It Matters:**
  Your monitor should be directly in front of you to avoid twisting your neck and back.

- **What to Do:**
  - Centre the monitor directly in front of you, so you don't have to turn your head to view the screen.

  - If using multiple monitors, place the primary monitor directly in front of you and the secondary monitor slightly to the side, but close enough that you can view it without excessive neck movement.

Keyboard and Mouse Placement

- **Keyboard Position**

- **Why It Matters:**
  Proper keyboard placement helps maintain a neutral wrist position and reduces strain on your arms, shoulders, and back.

- **What to Do:**
  - Place the keyboard directly in front of you, close enough that your elbows remain close to your body when typing.

  - Your forearms should be parallel to the floor, and your wrists should be in a neutral position (not bent up or down).

  - If necessary, use a keyboard tray that allows you to adjust the height and angle of the keyboard for comfort.

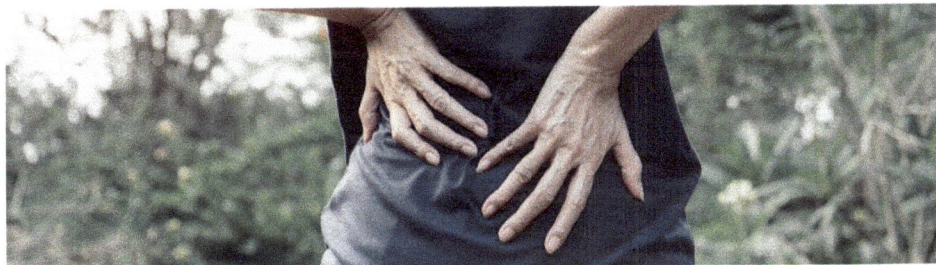

Mouse Placement

- **Why It Matters:**
The mouse should be placed close to the keyboard to prevent overreaching, which can strain your shoulder and back.

- **What to Do:**
  - Position the mouse at the same level as the keyboard, within easy reach.

  - Keep your wrist in a neutral position while using the mouse and use your whole arm to move the mouse rather than just your wrist.

Foot Placement

Footrest Use

- **Why It Matters:**
If your feet do not comfortably reach the floor, a footrest can help maintain proper posture and reduce strain on your lower back.

- **What to Do:**
  - Use a footrest if your chair is adjusted higher to accommodate the desk height, ensuring your feet are flat and supported.

  - Your feet should be flat on the footrest, with your knees at a 90-degree angle.

Lighting and Screen Glare

Proper Lighting

- **Why It Matters:**
Good lighting reduces eye strain, which can indirectly affect your posture and contribute to back and neck discomfort.

- **What to Do:**
  - Position your desk in a well-lit area, preferably with natural light. Use task lighting if needed to reduce screen glare.

  - Adjust your monitor's brightness and contrast to reduce strain on your eyes.

Screen Glare Reduction

- **Why It Matters:**
  Glare on the screen can cause you to adjust your posture to see better, leading to strain on your neck and back.

- **What to Do:**
  - Position your monitor to minimise glare from windows or overhead lights.

  - Use an anti-glare screen or adjust blinds and lighting to reduce glare.

Taking Breaks and Movement

Frequent Breaks

- **Why It Matters:**
  Sitting for prolonged periods can lead to stiffness and back pain. Regular breaks help maintain circulation and reduce muscle tension.

- **What to Do:**
  - Take short breaks every 30-60 minutes to stand, stretch, and walk around.

  - Consider using a timer or time application to remind you to take breaks throughout the day.

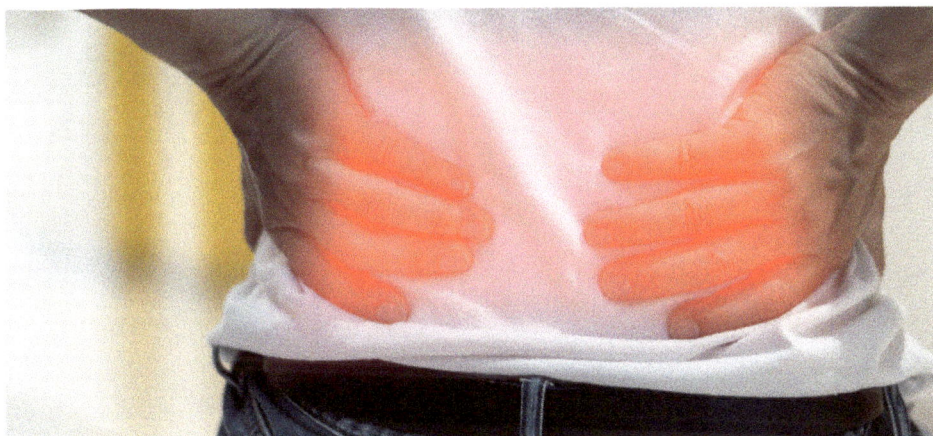

Desk Ergonomics

- **Why It Matters:**
  A well-organised and ergonomic desk setup can help you maintain good posture and reduce the risk of back strain.

- **What to Do:**
  - Keep your workspace clean and organised to minimise reaching and awkward movements.

  - Use ergonomic accessories, such as a document holder or phone stand, to keep items at eye level and within easy reach.

Setting up your desk and computer is essential for minimising back strain and promoting good posture. By paying attention to the height and placement of your chair, monitor, keyboard, and other workspace elements, you can create an ergonomic environment that supports your back health and overall well-being. Regular breaks and adjustments to your posture throughout the day are also crucial in preventing back pain. If you experience persistent discomfort, consider consulting an ergonomic specialist, occupational therapist or physical therapist for personalised advice and adjustments.

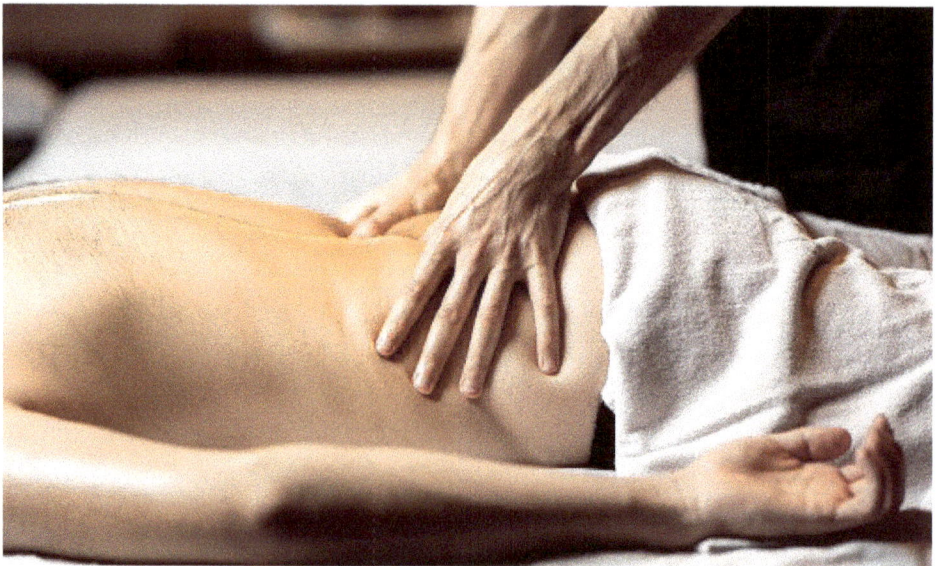

WHAT IS THE CORRECT POSTURE I SHOULD MAINTAIN WHILE SITTING FOR LONG PERIODS?

Maintaining correct posture while sitting for long periods is crucial for preventing back pain and reducing strain on your spine, neck, and shoulders. Good sitting posture helps distribute your body weight evenly, supports the natural curves of your spine, and minimises the risk of developing musculoskeletal issues. Here's a detailed guide on the correct posture to maintain while sitting for extended periods:

Key Elements of Correct Sitting Posture

Feet Placement

- **What to Do:**
  - Keep your feet flat on the floor, with your knees bent at a 90-degree angle.

  - If your feet don't reach the floor comfortably, use a footrest to support them.

- **Why It Matters:**
  Proper foot placement helps maintain stability and prevents strain on your lower back and hips.

Knee and Hip Alignment

- **What to Do:**
  - Your knees should be at the same level as, or slightly lower than, your hips.

  - Maintain a 90-degree angle between your thighs and lower legs.

- **Why It Matters:**
  This alignment helps reduce pressure on your lower back and promotes proper circulation in your legs.

Use of a Supportive Chair

- **What to Do:**
  - Sit in a chair that provides firm support for your lower back and encourages an upright posture.

  - The backrest should support the natural curve of your lower spine (lumbar region).

- **Why It Matters:**
  A supportive chair helps maintain the natural curve of your spine and reduces the risk of slouching or leaning forward.

Back Position

- **What to Do:**
  - Sit with your back straight and shoulders relaxed, with your back fully supported by the chair's backrest.

  - Use a lumbar cushion or roll if your chair doesn't provide adequate lower back support.

- **Why It Matters:**
  Maintaining an upright back position helps distribute your body weight evenly and reduces the strain on your spine and back muscles.

Shoulder and Neck Alignment

- **What to Do:**
  - Keep your shoulders relaxed and avoid hunching them forward.

  - Your ears should be in line with your shoulders, and your head should be centred over your spine.

- **Why It Matters:**
  Proper shoulder and neck alignment reduces tension in the upper back, shoulders, and neck, and prevents the development of "tech neck" or forward head posture.

Arm and Elbow Position

- **What to Do:**
  - Keep your elbows close to your body and bent at a 90-degree angle when typing or using a mouse.

  - Your forearms should be parallel to the floor, with your wrists in a neutral position (not bent up or down).

- **Why It Matters:**
  Proper arm and elbow positioning reduces strain on your shoulders, arms, and wrists, helping to prevent repetitive strain injuries.

Wrist and Hand Position

- **What to Do:**
  - Keep your wrists straight and in line with your forearms while typing or using a mouse.

  - Use a wrist rest if needed to maintain a neutral wrist position.

- **Why It Matters:**
  Maintaining a neutral wrist position helps prevent carpal tunnel syndrome and reduces strain on your forearms.

Head and Eye Level

- **What to Do:**
  - Position your computer monitor at eye level, about an arm's length away, so you can look straight ahead without tilting your head up or down.

  - If you use multiple monitors, ensure the primary monitor is directly in front of you, and adjust the height and angle as needed..

- **Why It Matters:**
  Proper head and eye alignment reduces the risk of neck strain and helps maintain good posture.

Additional Tips for Maintaining Good Sitting Posture

Take Regular Breaks

- **What to Do:**
  Stand up, stretch, and walk around every 30-60 minutes to relieve pressure on your back and improve circulation.

- **Why It Matters:**
  Regular movement helps prevent stiffness and muscle fatigue, which can develop from sitting for extended periods.

Adjust Your Position Frequently

- **What to Do:**
  Shift your sitting position slightly throughout the day to distribute pressure and avoid overloading any specific muscle group.

- **Why It Matters:**
  Regular adjustments help prevent muscle strain and discomfort that can result from holding a static position for too long.

Use Ergonomic Accessories

- **What to Do:**
  Consider using ergonomic accessories, such as a lumbar roll, footrest, or ergonomic keyboard and mouse, to enhance your comfort and support proper posture.

- **Why It Matters:**
  Ergonomic tools can help you maintain good posture and reduce the risk of developing musculoskeletal issues.

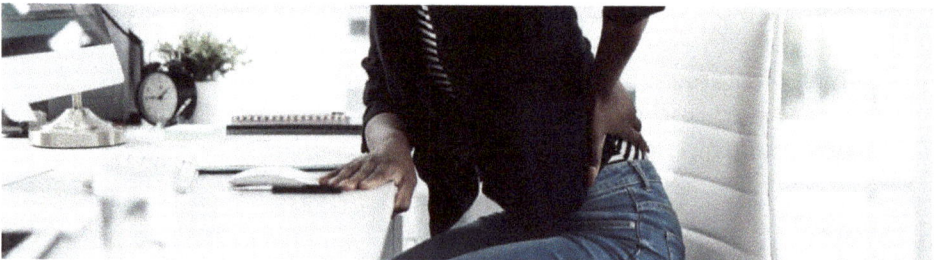

Mind Your Posture When Leaning Forward

- **What to Do:**
  If you need to lean forward to perform a task, do so from your hips rather than rounding your back. Keep your spine straight and engage your core muscles.

- **Why It Matters:**
  Leaning forward incorrectly can lead to poor posture and back strain, so it's important to maintain proper alignment even when reaching forward.

Maintaining correct posture while sitting for prolonged periods is essential for preventing back pain and reducing strain on your spine and muscles. By following the guidelines above and by focusing on proper alignment of your feet, knees, hips, back, shoulders, neck, and arms you can minimise the risk of developing musculoskeletal issues and improve your overall comfort.

Incorporating regular breaks, using ergonomic accessories, and making small adjustments to your posture throughout the day will further support your back health. If you experience persistent discomfort or pain despite maintaining good posture, consider consulting a healthcare provider or physical therapist for further advice and adjustments to your sitting setup.

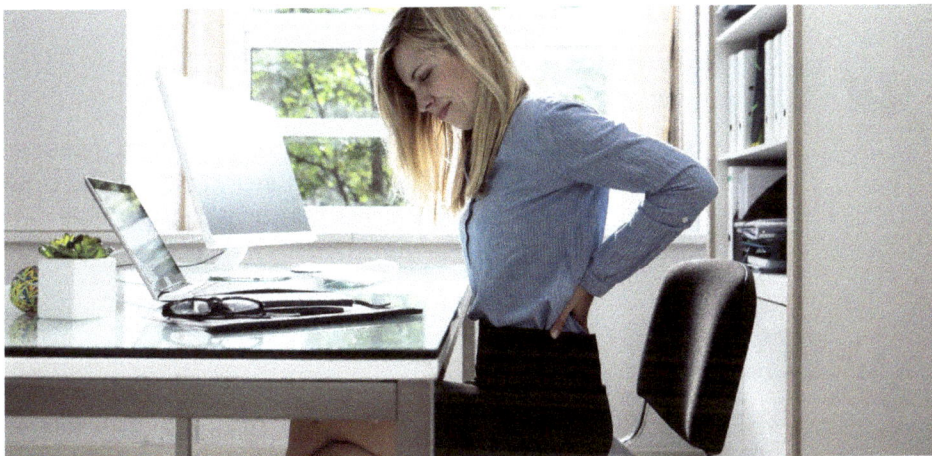

SHOULD I USE A STANDING DESK, AND HOW DO I SET IT UP PROPERLY TO AVOID BACK PAIN?

Should You Use a Standing Desk?

Using a standing desk can offer several benefits, especially if you spend long hours sitting. Alternating between sitting and standing throughout the day can help reduce the risk of back pain, improve posture, and increase overall comfort. However, it's important to set up a standing desk properly and use it correctly to avoid introducing new strains or discomfort.

Benefits of Using a Standing Desk

Reduced Back Pain

Alternating between sitting and standing can reduce the strain on your lower back, hips, and spine by promoting better posture and encouraging movement.

Improved Posture

Standing desks can help you maintain a more neutral spine alignment, reducing the likelihood of slouching or hunching over.

Increased Energy and Focus

Many people report feeling more energetic and focused when they stand part of the day, as standing encourages more movement and reduces the lethargy associated with prolonged sitting

Better Circulation

Standing increases blood flow and reduces the risk of circulation issues that can occur with prolonged sitting.

How to Set Up a Standing Desk Properly to Avoid Back Pain

Adjust Desk Height Correctly

- **How to Do It:**
  - The desk height should be set so that your elbows are at a 90-degree angle when your forearms are parallel to the desk surface.

  - Your wrists should remain in a neutral position, not bent up or down, while typing.

- **Why It Matters:**
  Proper desk height helps maintain neutral wrist alignment and reduces strain on your arms, shoulders, and back.

Monitor Position

- **How to Do It:**
  - Position your monitor at eye level so that the top of the screen is at or slightly below eye height.

  - The monitor should be about an arm's length away, allowing you to view the screen without leaning forward or straining your neck.

- **Why It Matters:**
  Correct monitor placement helps maintain proper neck and head alignment, reducing the risk of neck and upper back pain.

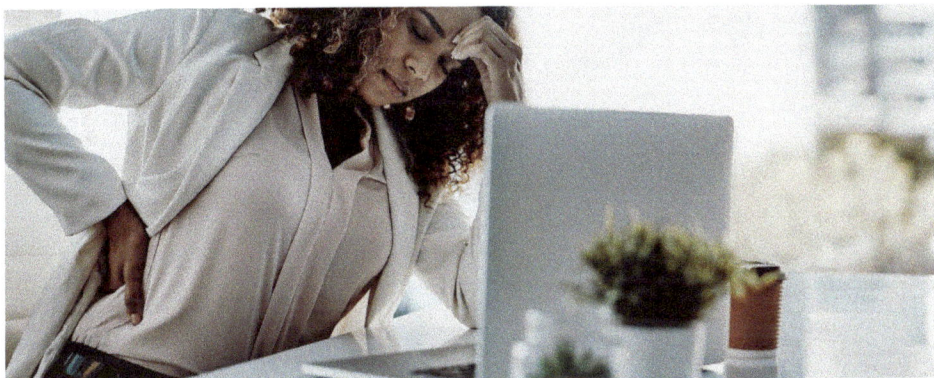

Footwear and Floor Surface

- **How to Do It:**
  - Wear supportive shoes that provide good arch support and cushioning.

  - Consider using an anti-fatigue mat if you're standing on a hard surface, as it can reduce pressure on your feet and lower back.

- **Why It Matters:**
  Supportive footwear and proper floor cushioning help prevent foot, leg, and lower back discomfort when standing for extended periods.

Foot Placement and Posture

- **How to Do It:**
  - Stand with your feet shoulder-width apart and distribute your weight evenly between both feet.

  - Keep your knees slightly bent rather than locking them to maintain a natural standing posture.

  - Engage your core muscles to support your lower back and avoid slouching or leaning on one leg.

- **Why It Matters:**
  Proper foot placement and posture help maintain spinal alignment and reduce the risk of back pain.

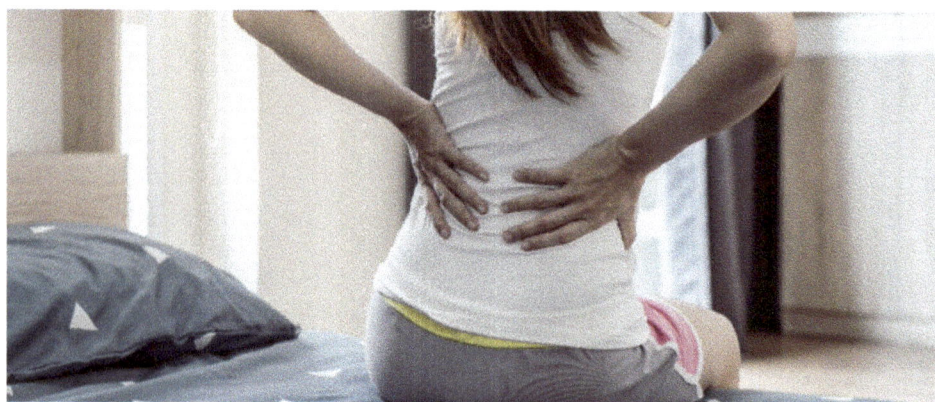

Alternate Between Sitting and Standing

- **How to Do It:**
  - Alternate between sitting and standing every 30-60 minutes to prevent muscle fatigue and reduce strain on your back and legs.

  - Use a sit-stand desk converter or an adjustable standing desk to easily switch between positions.

- **Why It Matters:**
  Alternating between sitting and standing helps avoid the strain associated with prolonged sitting or standing and promotes overall comfort and productivity.

Use Ergonomic Accessories

- **How to Do It:**
  - Consider using a footrest to shift your weight and relieve pressure on your lower back.

  - Use an ergonomic keyboard and mouse to maintain proper wrist alignment.

  - If your standing desk's chair (bar stool like) doesn't have built-in lumbar support, consider using a small cushion or lumbar roll to support your lower back when sitting.

- **Why It Matters:**
  Ergonomic accessories enhance comfort and support proper posture while using a standing desk, reducing the risk of strain and injury.

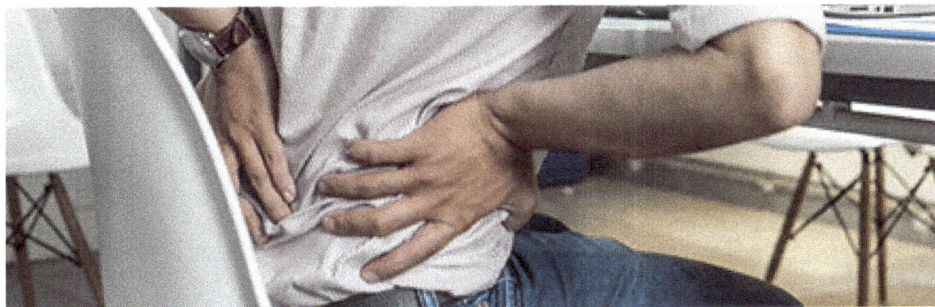

Monitor Your Body's Response

- **How to Do It:**
  - Pay attention to how your body feels throughout the day. If you experience discomfort or fatigue, adjust your posture, desk height, or take a break to sit or move around.

- **Why It Matters:**
  Listening to your body helps you make necessary adjustments to prevent strain and maintain comfort while using a standing desk.

Tips for Transitioning to a Standing Desk

1. **Start Slowly:**
   If you're new to using a standing desk, start by standing for short periods and gradually increase the duration as your body adapts. Aim to stand for 15-30 minutes at a time and gradually work up to longer periods.

2. **Incorporate Movement:**
   Don't stand still for extended periods. Shift your weight from one foot to the other, move around, and take breaks to walk or stretch. This helps prevent stiffness and promotes circulation.

3. **Use a Chair for Sitting Breaks:**
   Have a comfortable chair nearby so you can switch between sitting and standing throughout the day. An ergonomic chair with good lumbar support is ideal for sitting breaks.

   A modified "bar stool" can be useful for "sitting" as can support the pelvis while standing.

4. **Stretch Regularly:**
   Incorporate regular stretching into your routine to relieve tension and maintain flexibility. Stretch your back, legs, and shoulders to prevent stiffness.

Using a standing desk can be beneficial for preventing and managing back pain, but it's essential to set it up correctly and use it wisely. By paying attention to desk height, monitor placement, posture, and ergonomics, you can reduce the risk of strain and discomfort. Remember to alternate between sitting and standing, use supportive footwear, and incorporate movement throughout the day to stay comfortable and maintain good back health.

If you experience persistent discomfort while using a standing desk, consider consulting with an ergonomic specialist for advice.

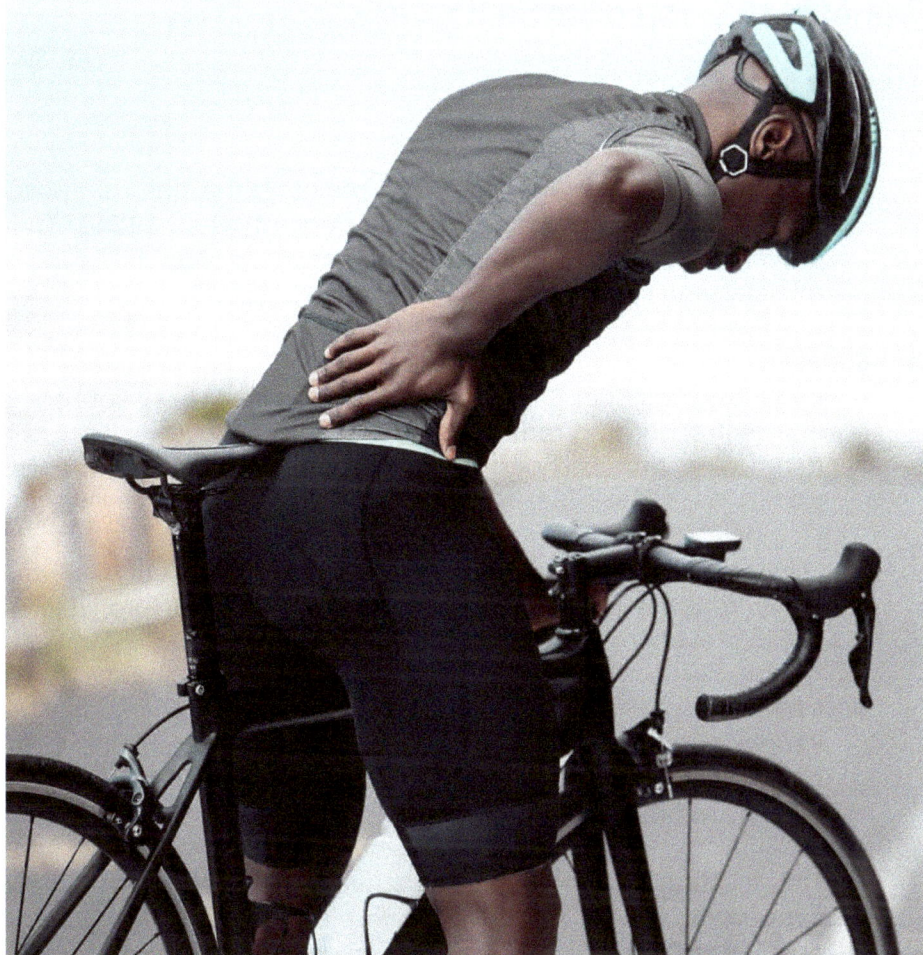

DO I NEED TO USE ERGONOMIC ACCESSORIES (LIKE LUMBAR SUPPORTS OR FOOTRESTS) TO HELP WITH BACK PAIN?

Using ergonomic accessories such as lumbar supports, footrests, and other ergonomic tools can be highly beneficial in preventing and managing back pain, especially if you spend extended periods sitting or standing at work. These accessories are designed to promote good posture, reduce strain on your back, and support the natural alignment of your spine. Here's how different ergonomic accessories can help and whether you might need them:

Benefits of Using a Standing Desk

Lumbar Support

- **What It Does:**
  - Lumbar supports are designed to maintain the natural inward curve of your lower spine (lumbar region) when sitting. They prevent slouching and reduce the strain on your lower back muscles and spinal discs.

- **Benefits:**
  - Reduces Lower Back Strain: Lumbar support helps keep your spine in a neutral position, reducing the pressure on the lower back and decreasing the likelihood of developing or exacerbating back pain.

  - Promotes Good Posture: By supporting the natural curve of your spine, lumbar supports encourage proper sitting posture, which is key to preventing back pain.

- **Who Needs It:**
  - People with Existing Back Pain: If you already experience lower back pain, a lumbar support cushion can provide immediate relief by reducing pressure on your spine.

  - Those Sitting for Long Periods: If your chair lacks built-in lumbar support or if you sit for extended periods, using a lumbar cushion can help maintain proper spinal alignment and prevent discomfort.

- **Types of Lumbar Support:**
  - Built-in Lumbar Support: Some office chairs come with adjustable lumbar support built into the backrest. If your chair has this feature, adjust it to fit the natural curve of your spine.

  - External Lumbar Cushions: If your chair doesn't have built-in support, you can use an external lumbar cushion or roll to provide the necessary support.

Footrests

- **What It Does:**
  - Footrests elevate your feet slightly, helping to maintain a 90-degree angle at your knees and hips, which supports proper posture.

- **Benefits:**
  - Improves Posture: A footrest helps ensure that your feet are flat and supported, which can prevent slouching and reduce strain on your lower back and legs.

  - Reduces Pressure on Lower Back: By elevating your feet, a footrest can reduce pressure on your lower back, especially if your chair height doesn't allow your feet to rest comfortably on the floor.

- **Who Needs It:**
  - Shorter Individuals: If your feet don't reach the floor comfortably when sitting, a footrest is essential to maintain proper posture and reduce strain.

  - Those with Circulation Issues: A footrest can also help improve circulation by preventing your legs from dangling or being compressed against the seat.

- **Types of Footrests:**
  - Adjustable Footrests: Look for footrests with adjustable height and angle settings to find the most comfortable position.

  - Non-Slip Footrests: A footrest with a non-slip surface helps keep your feet in place and prevents the accessory from sliding around.

Wrist Rests

- **What It Does:**
  - Wrist rests support your wrists while typing or using a mouse, helping to maintain a neutral wrist position.

- **Benefits:**
  - Reduces Strain on Wrists and Forearms: Wrist rests help prevent your wrists from bending upwards or downwards, which can reduce strain and the risk of developing conditions like carpal tunnel syndrome.

  - Improves Comfort: They provide cushioning and support, making it more comfortable to work for extended periods.

- **Who Needs It:**
  - Frequent Computer Users: If you spend a lot of time typing or using a mouse, wrist rests can help reduce the strain on your wrists and forearms.

- **Types of Footrests:**
  - Keyboard Wrist Rests: These are placed in front of the keyboard to support your wrists while typing.

  - Mouse Wrist Rests: These are used alongside your mouse to maintain wrist alignment during mouse movements

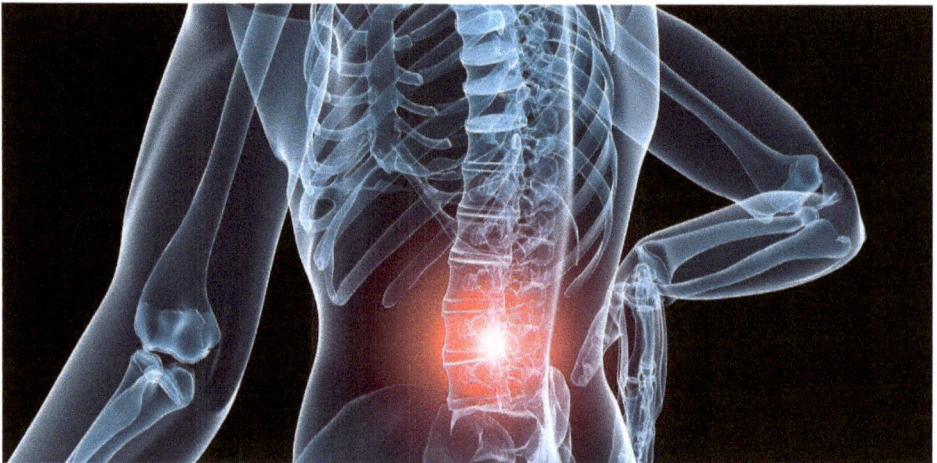

Ergonomic Keyboard and Mouse

- **What It Does:**
  - Ergonomic keyboards and mice are designed to reduce strain on your hands, wrists, and arms by promoting a more natural hand position.

- **Benefits:**
  - Reduces Strain: Ergonomic keyboards often have a split design that allows your hands to rest in a more natural position, reducing strain on your wrists and forearms.

  - Promotes Comfort: An ergonomic mouse supports the natural curve of your hand, reducing tension in your fingers and wrist.

- **Who Needs It:**
  - People with Repetitive Strain Injuries (RSIs): If you experience discomfort or have a history of RSIs, an ergonomic keyboard and mouse can help alleviate symptoms.

  - Those with Extended Computer Use: Anyone who spends long hours on the computer can benefit from the improved comfort and reduced strain provided by ergonomic devices.

Monitor Stands

- **What It Does:**
  - Monitor stands elevate your computer screen to eye level, helping to prevent neck and upper back strain.

- **Benefits:**
  - Promotes Proper Neck Alignment: Keeping your monitor at eye level helps maintain a neutral neck position and prevents forward head posture.

  - Reduces Eye Strain: Proper monitor height can also help reduce eye strain by ensuring you're looking straight ahead rather than up or down.

- **Who Needs It:**
  - People with Improper Monitor Height: If your monitor is too low or too high, a stand can help position it correctly to avoid strain.

  - Dual Monitor Users: If you use multiple monitors, stands can help ensure all screens are at the correct height and angle.

Ergonomic accessories like lumbar supports, footrests, and other tools can be highly effective in preventing and managing back pain by promoting proper posture and reducing strain on your body by helping the shock absorption. Whether you need these accessories depends on your specific situation, including your existing setup, the duration of your sitting or standing, and any current discomfort or back pain you're experiencing.

If you frequently experience back pain or discomfort, it's a good idea to consider incorporating these ergonomic accessories into your workspace. They can provide immediate relief and contribute to long-term spinal health. However, it's important to choose accessories that are well-suited to your individual needs and to adjust them properly for maximum benefit. If you're unsure about what you need, consulting with an ergonomic specialist or a healthcare provider can help you create an optimised workspace that supports your health and comfort.

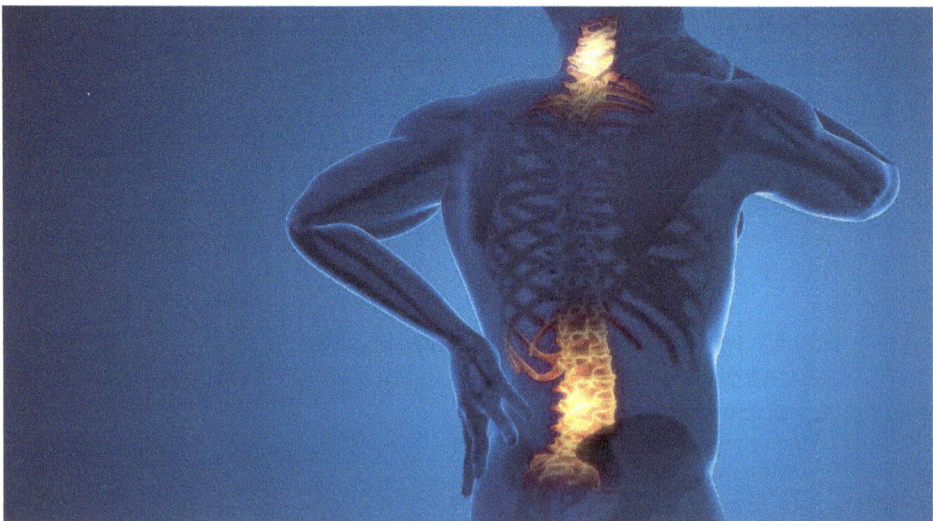

HOW OFTEN SHOULD I TAKE BREAKS TO STRETCH OR MOVE AROUND IF I AM REQUIRED TO SIT FOR EXTENDED PERIODS?

After sitting for extended periods, it's essential to take regular breaks to stretch and move around to prevent back pain, stiffness, and other health issues. Here's a guideline on how often you should take breaks and what you can do during these breaks:

How Often Should You Take Breaks?
Every 30 Minutes

- **What to Do:**
  Ideally, you should take a brief break to stand up, stretch, or move around every 30 minutes.

- **Why It Matters:**
  Sitting for extended periods can lead to muscle stiffness, reduced circulation, and increased strain on your back and spine. Regular breaks help mitigate these effects.

The 20-20-20 Rule

- **What to Do:**
  For eye strain prevention, follow the 20-20-20 rule: every 20 minutes, look at something 20 feet away for at least 20 seconds. This can also serve as a reminder to adjust your posture or stand up.

- **Why It Matters:**
  This rule primarily helps prevent eye strain, but it also encourages regular intervals for movement or posture adjustment.

Hourly Movement

- **What to Do:**
  At least once every hour, take a slightly longer break (3-5 minutes) to walk around, do some stretches, or change your position.

- **Why It Matters:**
  This helps prevent the negative effects of prolonged sitting, such as decreased circulation and muscle fatigue

What to Do During Breaks

Lumbar Support

Stretching Exercises:
- Neck Stretch: Gently tilt your head toward each shoulder, holding for 15-20 seconds on each side to stretch the neck muscles.

- Shoulder Rolls: Roll your shoulders backward and forward in a circular motion to relieve tension in your shoulders and upper back.

- Chest Stretch: Interlace your fingers behind your back and gently pull your shoulders back and down to open up the chest and stretch the front of your shoulders.

- Back Extension: Stand up, place your hands on your lower back, and gently arch your back, looking up at the ceiling. Hold for 10-15 seconds to stretch your lower back.

- Hamstring Stretch: While standing, place one foot on a low stool or chair, keeping your leg straight, and gently lean forward to stretch your hamstring.

Movement:
- Walking: Take a short walk around your office or home to get your blood flowing and relieve stiffness in your legs and lower back.

- Marching in Place: If you can't leave your workstation, march in place for a minute to engage your leg muscles and promote circulation.

- Leg Swings: Stand and hold onto a stable surface for balance, then gently swing one leg forward and backward to loosen up your hip flexors.

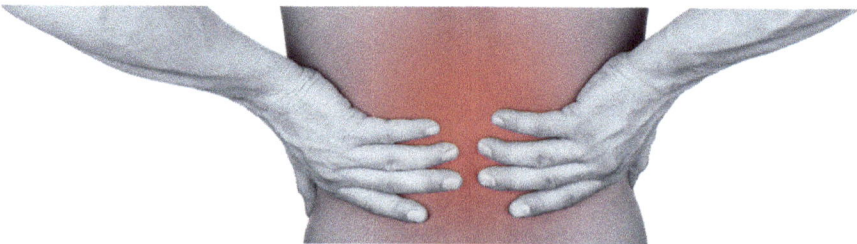

Posture Reset:
- Reassess Your Posture: After each break, return to your chair and reassess your sitting posture. Make sure your back is straight, shoulders are relaxed, and feet are flat on the floor.

- Adjust Your Chair: If needed, adjust your chair's height or lumbar support to maintain a comfortable sitting position.

Hydration:
- Drink Water: Use your breaks to drink water. Staying hydrated is important for overall health and can also encourage you to take more breaks, as you'll need to get up to refill your glass or visit the restroom.

- Why It Matters: Proper hydration supports circulation and can help reduce muscle cramps and fatigue.

Why Regular Breaks Are Important

Prevents Muscle Fatigue

Regular movement prevents your muscles from becoming fatigued and stiff, which can lead to discomfort and pain.

Improves Circulation

Moving around promotes blood flow, which is essential for delivering oxygen and nutrients to your muscles and preventing the formation of blood clots.

Reduces Strain on the Spine

Regular movement prevents your muscles from becoming fatigued and stiff, which can lead to discomfort and pain.

Enhances Mental Focus

Regular movement prevents your muscles from becoming fatigued and stiff, which can lead to discomfort and pain.

To prevent back pain and other health issues associated with prolonged sitting, it's recommended to take brief breaks every 30 minutes, follow the 20-20-20 rule for eye strain, and incorporate slightly longer movement breaks every hour. During these breaks, perform stretches, move around, and reassess your posture to keep your body and mind refreshed.

By making regular breaks a habit, you can significantly reduce the negative effects of long periods of sitting and support your overall health and well-being. If you find it difficult to remember to take breaks, consider using a timer, break reminder app, or setting calendar alerts to prompt you throughout the day.

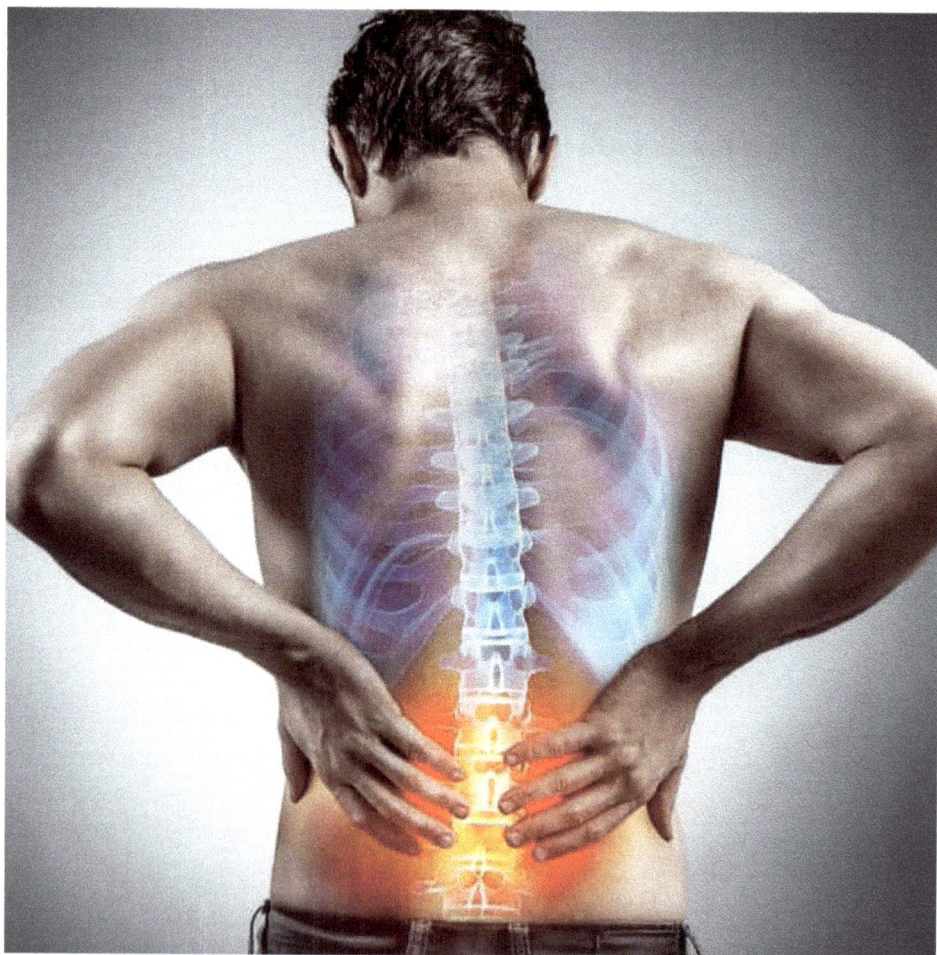

WHAT IS THE BEST WAY TO LIFT HEAVY OBJECTS TO AVOID BACK STRAIN?

Lifting heavy objects incorrectly is a common cause of back strain and injury. To avoid back strain, it's important to use proper lifting techniques that protect your spine and distribute the load evenly across your body. Here's a step-by-step guide on the best way to lift heavy objects safely:

Understanding

Assess the Load
Evaluate the Weight:
- Before lifting, test the weight of the object by pushing it slightly with your foot or hands. If it feels too heavy, seek help or use equipment like a dolly or hand truck.

- **Plan Your Route:**
  - Ensure the path to your destination is clear of obstacles and that you have a clear space to set the object down

Action

Position Yourself Properly
Stand Close to the Object:
- Position yourself as close to the object as possible. The closer the object is to your body, the less strain it puts on your back.

Feet Placement:
- Place your feet shoulder-width apart to provide a stable base of support. One foot can be slightly ahead of the other to maintain balance.

Bend Your Knees and Hips
Bend at the Knees and Hips:
- Squat down by bending your knees and hips, not your waist. Keep your back straight (not rounded) throughout the movement.

Engage Your Core:
- Tighten your abdominal muscles as you squat down. Engaging your core helps support your spine and maintain proper posture.

Grip the Object Securely
Get a Firm Grip:
- Use both hands to securely grip the object. Ensure your grip is firm and the object is balanced.

Engage Your Core:
- Hold the object close to your body, ideally at the level of your belly button or slightly below. This reduces the strain on your back.

Lift with Your Legs
Use Your Leg Muscles:
- Lift the object by straightening your knees and hips, using the strength of your leg muscles rather than your back. Your back should remain straight as you lift.

Avoid Twisting:
- Keep your torso facing forward. Avoid twisting your back or turning your body while lifting, as this can increase the risk of injury. If you need to turn, pivot with your feet instead of twisting your back.

Carry the Load Safely
Maintain Proper Posture:
- As you carry the object, keep your back straight, shoulders back, and head up. Walk slowly and carefully, keeping the object close to your body.

Avoid Overreaching:
- Don't attempt to lift or carry objects above shoulder height. If you need to place an object on a high shelf, use a step stool or ladder.

Set the Object Down Carefully
Lower the Load with Your Legs:
- When you reach your destination, squat down by bending your knees and hips to lower the object. Keep your back straight and the object close to your body.

Place the Object Gently:
- Set the object down gently and in a controlled manner, avoiding any sudden or jerky movements.

Assistance

Seek Assistance When Needed
Use Team Lifting:
- If the object is too heavy or awkward to lift on your own, ask for help from a colleague or friend. Coordinate your movements to lift and carry the object together.

Use Mechanical Aids:
- For very heavy or bulky items, use mechanical aids such as dollies, hand trucks, or lifting straps to reduce the risk of injury.

Additional Tips for Safe Lifting

Warm Up
- Before lifting heavy objects, it's a good idea to do some light stretching or warm-up exercises to prepare your muscles for the task.

Wear Supportive Footwear
- Wear shoes with good traction and support to help maintain balance and stability while lifting.

Listen to Your Body
- If you feel any pain or discomfort while lifting, stop immediately. Pain is a sign that something is wrong, and continuing to lift could lead to injury.

Using proper lifting techniques is essential for avoiding back strain and injury when handling heavy objects. By positioning yourself correctly, using your leg muscles to lift, and keeping the load close to your body, you can significantly reduce the risk of back pain. Always remember to assess the load and seek assistance if needed. Regularly practicing these techniques will help protect your back and promote long-term spinal health.

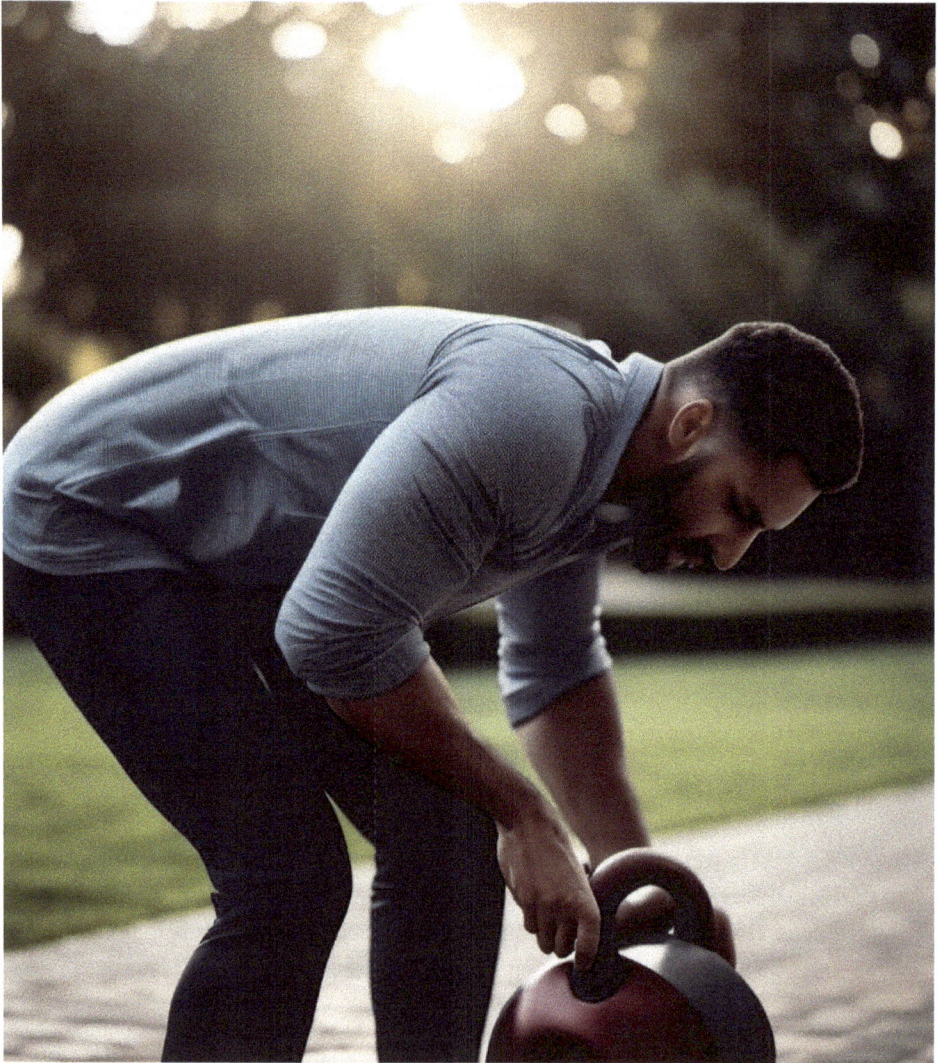

CAN AN ERGONOMIC KEYBOARD AND MOUSE HELP REDUCE BACK PAIN, AND HOW SHOULD THEY BE POSITIONED?

An ergonomic keyboard and mouse and can help reduce back pain, particularly when they are part of an overall ergonomic workstation setup. While these devices are primarily designed to reduce strain on your hands, wrists, and arms, they can indirectly benefit your back by promoting better posture and reducing tension throughout your body.

How an ergonomic Keyboard and Mouse Help

Promote Neutral Posture

An ergonomic keyboard and mouse are designed to promote a more natural, neutral posture for your hands and arms, which can prevent you from hunching over or adopting awkward positions that strain your back.

Reduce Muscle Tension

By minimising strain on your hands, wrists, and forearms, ergonomic devices reduce the overall tension in your upper body, which can translate into less strain on your shoulders, neck, and back.

Encourage Proper Alignment

Properly positioned ergonomic devices encourage you to sit with your shoulders relaxed and your back straight, which supports the natural curve of your spine and helps prevent back pain.

Positioning Ergonomic Keyboards

Height
- Position the Keyboard: The keyboard should be placed at a height where your forearms are parallel to the floor or slightly angled downward. Your elbows should be at a 90-degree angle, close to your body.

- Avoid Wrist Flexion: Your wrists should be in a neutral position, not bent upward or downward. If necessary, use a keyboard tray or an adjustable desk to achieve the correct height.

Distance
- Close Enough to Reach Comfortably: The keyboard should be close enough to your body so that you don't have to stretch your arms forward to type. Ideally, the keyboard should be placed just a few inches away from the edge of your desk.

Tilt
- Flat or Negative Tilt: The keyboard should be either flat or slightly tilted away from you (negative tilt). This position helps maintain a neutral wrist position and reduces the risk of wrist strain.

Split and Adjustable Keyboards
- Split Design: Some ergonomic keyboards are split into two halves, allowing you to position each half at an angle that suits your natural hand and wrist position. This design reduces ulnar deviation (the bending of the wrist towards the little finger), which can strain the wrists and forearms.

- Adjustable Angle and Tenting: Many ergonomic keyboards offer adjustable angles and tenting (a slight upward curve) to further reduce strain on your wrists and forearms.

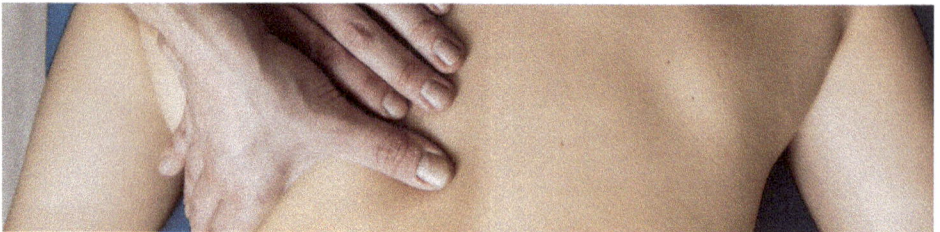

Positioning an ergonomic Mouse

Height
- Same Height as Keyboard: The mouse should be at the same height as your keyboard, ensuring that your forearm remains parallel to the floor while using it.

Distance
- Close to the Keyboard: Place the mouse as close to the keyboard as possible to minimise reaching. This reduces strain on your shoulder and upper back.

- Avoid Overreaching: Ensure that you don't have to extend your arm too far to use the mouse, as this can lead to shoulder and upper back pain.

Grip and Movement
- Relaxed Grip: Use a relaxed grip on the mouse, avoiding excessive pressure or tension in your hand and fingers.

- Use Your Arm, Not Just Your Wrist: When moving the mouse, try to use your arm rather than just your wrist. This reduces strain on the wrist and promotes better overall posture.

Vertical or Trackball Mouse
- Vertical Mouse: These are designed to keep your hand in a handshake position, which can reduce strain on your wrist and forearm muscles.

- Trackball Mouse: A trackball mouse allows you to control the cursor by rotating the ball with your fingers, reducing the need for wrist and arm movements.

Additional Ergonomic Considerations

Monitor Position
- At Eye Level: Ensure that your monitor is positioned at eye level and directly in front of you. This reduces the need to tilt your head up or down and helps maintain proper neck and back alignment.

- Distance: The monitor should be about an arm's length away, allowing you to see the screen clearly without leaning forward.

Chair and Posture

*   Supportive Chair: Use a chair with good lumbar support to maintain the natural curve of your spine.

*   Posture: Sit with your back straight, shoulders relaxed, and feet flat on the floor. Keep your elbows close to your body and avoid hunching over or leaning forward.

Breaks and Movement

*   Regular Breaks: Take regular breaks to stretch and move around. This helps reduce muscle tension and prevents the development of strain from prolonged sitting or repetitive motions.

An ergonomic keyboard and mouse can play a significant role in reducing back pain by promoting better posture and reducing strain on your hands, wrists, and arms. Properly positioning these devices is key to achieving their full ergonomic benefits. By ensuring that your keyboard and mouse are at the correct height, distance, and angle, and by using them in conjunction with an overall ergonomic workstation setup, you can minimise the risk of back pain and improve your overall comfort while working.

Use a specialist consultant on ergonomics if necessary.

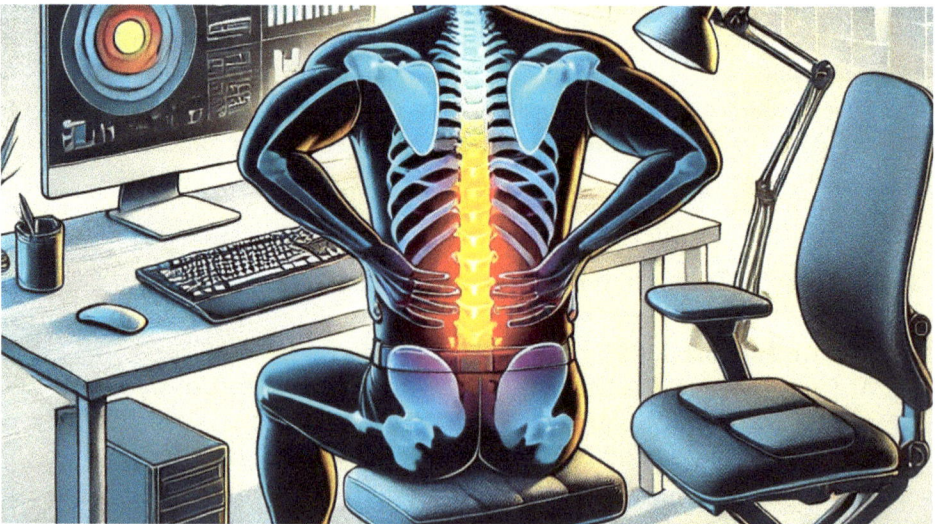

IS IT IMPORTANT TO HAVE AN ERGONOMIC MATTRESS OR PILLOW, AND HOW DO I CHOOSE THE RIGHT ONE?

Having an ergonomic mattress and pillow is crucial for maintaining proper spinal alignment and ensuring restful sleep, which are both essential for preventing and alleviating back pain. The right mattress and pillow support the natural curves of your spine, reducing pressure points and minimising the risk of discomfort or pain during sleep.

Choosing the Right Ergonomic Mattress
Support and Firmness
- Medium-Firm: A medium-firm mattress is often recommended because it provides adequate support for your spine while still offering enough cushioning for comfort. This balance helps keep your spine in a neutral position.

- Personal Preference: While a medium firm is recommended, the best mattress firmness can vary based on your body weight, sleep position, and personal comfort preferences. Heavier individuals might prefer a firmer mattress for better support, while lighter individuals might find a softer mattress more comfortable.

Mattress Type
- Memory Foam: Memory foam mattresses contour to your body shape, providing customised support and relieving pressure points. They are particularly good for side sleepers as they cushion the shoulders and hips.

- Latex: Latex mattresses are durable and offer a good balance of support and comfort. They are responsive and slightly firmer than memory foam, making them a good option for back and stomach sleepers.

- Innerspring: Innerspring mattresses offer good support and are typically firmer. They can be a good option for those who prefer a more traditional feel, but it's important to choose one with adequate cushioning to prevent pressure points.

- Hybrid: Hybrid mattresses combine innerspring coils with foam or latex layers, offering a mix of support and comfort. They are versatile and can suit various sleeping positions.

Spinal Alignment
- Neutral Spine: When lying down, your mattress should support the natural curve of your spine. For side sleepers, your spine should remain straight, and for back sleepers, it should maintain its natural curve. Stomach sleeping is generally discouraged because it can strain the neck and lower back, but if you do sleep on your stomach, a firmer mattress is usually better to prevent sagging.

Pressure Relief
- Pressure Points: A good mattress should relieve pressure points, particularly at the hips, shoulders, and knees, depending on your sleeping position. Memory foam and latex are particularly good at distributing weight evenly to reduce pressure.

Durability and Longevity
- o Quality Materials: Invest in a high-quality mattress that offers durability and maintains its shape and support over time. A good mattress should last about 7-10 years.

Choosing the Right Ergonomic Pillow

Pillow Loft (Height)
- Side Sleepers: Side sleepers need a high-loft pillow that fills the space between the neck and the mattress, keeping the spine aligned. The pillow should be firm enough to support the neck but soft enough to conform to the shoulder.

- Back Sleepers: Back sleepers usually benefit from a medium-loft pillow that supports the natural curve of the neck without pushing the head too far forward. A contoured memory foam pillow can be particularly effective.

- Stomach Sleepers: Stomach sleepers need a low-loft pillow to prevent neck strain. Some stomach sleepers even prefer sleeping without a pillow or using a very thin pillow.

Pillow Material

- Memory Foam: Memory foam pillows conform to the shape of your head and neck, providing customised support. They are excellent for maintaining proper alignment, especially for side and back sleepers.

- Latex: Latex pillows are firm and supportive while still offering some contouring. They are durable and retain their shape well, making them a desirable choice for back and side sleepers.

- Feather/Down: Feather or down pillows are soft and mouldable, making them good for those who like to adjust their pillow's shape throughout the night. However, they may not provide consistent support for those with neck or back issues.

- Adjustable Pillows: Some pillows allow you to add or remove filling to adjust the loft and firmness, making them versatile for different sleep positions and preferences.

Neck and Shoulder Support

- Contour Pillows: Contoured pillows are designed to cradle the neck and keep the spine aligned, making them a good choice for those with chronic neck or shoulder pain.

- Cervical Pillows: These pillows are specifically designed to support the cervical spine (neck) and are often recommended for those with neck pain or injuries.

Allergies and Breathability:

- Hypoallergenic Materials: If you have allergies, choose a pillow made from hypoallergenic materials. Memory foam and latex are naturally resistant to dust mites.

- Breathability: Consider the breathability of the pillow material, especially if you tend to sleep hot. Some memory foam pillows come with cooling gel layers or breathable covers to enhance airflow.

Testing and Trial Periods

Test Before You Buy
- Whenever possible, test mattresses and pillows in-store to get a feel for their support and comfort. Lie down in your usual sleep position to see how well the product supports your body.

Test Before You Buy

Whenever possible, test mattresses and pillows in-store to get a feel for their support and comfort. Lie down in your usual sleep position to see how well the product supports your body.

Trial Periods

Many mattress companies offer trial periods, allowing you to test the mattress at home for a certain period (often 90-120 days). This gives you time to see how well the mattress supports your sleep and if it alleviates your back pain.

Investing in an ergonomic mattress and pillow is important for maintaining spinal alignment, reducing pressure points, and ensuring a restful night's sleep, all of which are crucial for preventing or alleviating back pain. The right choice depends on your sleep position, body type, and personal preferences. A medium-firm mattress works well for most people, while the pillow height and material should be tailored to your sleep position. Consider testing products in-store and taking advantage of trial periods to find the best fit for your needs. If you continue to experience discomfort or pain, consulting a healthcare professional or sleep specialist may help you identify the most appropriate bedding options for your situation.

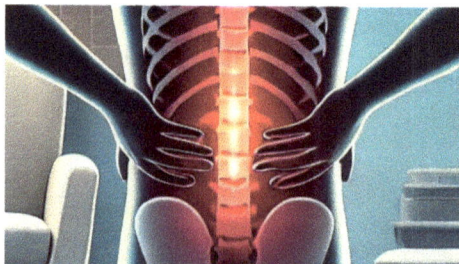

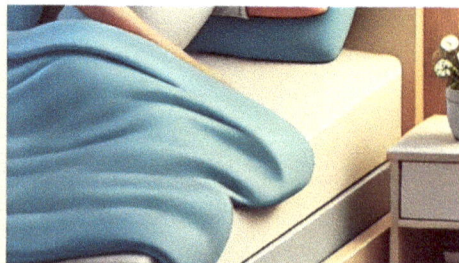

QUESTIONS ABOUT ERGONOMICS FOR PROFESSIONAL DRIVERS WHO SUFFER FROM BACK PAIN

These questions focus on the specific ergonomic adjustments and strategies that professional drivers can use to manage and alleviate back pain while spending extended periods in their vehicles.

HOW SHOULD I ADJUST MY SEAT TO PREVENT BACK PAIN DURING LONG DRIVES?

Adjusting your seat properly is essential for preventing back pain during long drives. A well-adjusted seat supports your spine's natural alignment, reduces muscle fatigue, and minimises strain on your back and neck. Here's how to adjust your seat for optimal comfort and back support:

Seat Height

Adjust the Seat Height

- Your seat should be high enough so that your hips are at the same level as, or slightly higher than, your knees. This position reduces strain on your lower back.

- Ensure that you have a clear view of the road and dashboard without needing to stretch or slouch.

- Your feet should comfortably reach the pedals, allowing you to press them fully without straining.

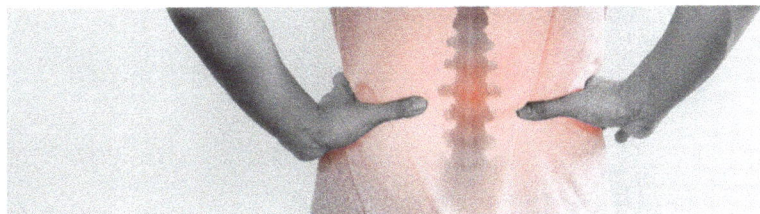

Seat Angle

Recline the Seat Slightly

- The seatback should be reclined at an angle of about 100 to 110 degrees. This slight recline helps maintain the natural curve of your lower spine (lumbar region) and reduces pressure on your discs.

- Avoid reclining too far back, as this can cause you to slouch and strain your neck and upper back.

Seat Distance from Pedals

Adjust the Seat Distance

- Position the seat so that you can reach the pedals comfortably with your knees slightly bent. Your legs should not be fully extended, as this can strain your lower back and hips.

- You should be able to press the pedals without having to lean forward, keeping your back in contact with the seatback.

Lumbar Support

Use Built-In Lumbar Support

- If your car seat has adjustable lumbar support, position it to fit the natural curve of your lower back. The lumbar support should fill the gap between your lower spine and the seatback, providing consistent support.

- External Lumbar Cushion: If your car seat doesn't have built-in lumbar support, consider using an external lumbar cushion or roll to support your lower back.

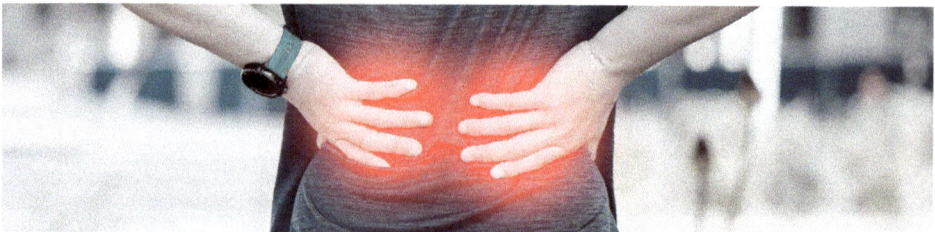

Seat Depth

Adjust Seat Depth (If Adjustable):
•   The seat cushion should support your thighs without putting pressure on the back of your knees. There should be about 2-3 inches (5-7 centimetres) of space between the edge of the seat and the back of your knees.

•   If your car seat has adjustable seat depth, set it to provide full thigh support while allowing free movement of your legs.

Headrest Position

Adjust the Headrest
•   The top of the headrest should be at least as high as the top of your head, and it should be positioned close to the back of your head (within about 2 inches or 5 centimetres).

•   The headrest should support the middle of the back of your head, helping to prevent neck strain and whiplash injuries in the event of a collision.

Steering Wheel Position

Adjust the Steering Wheel
•   Position the steering wheel so that you can hold it comfortably with your arms slightly bent at about a 120-degree angle.

•   The steering wheel should be close enough that you can reach it without stretching, but far enough that there is a gap of about 10-12 inches between your chest and the wheel.

•   Adjust the tilt of the steering wheel so that your hands are in a comfortable position, usually at the 9 and 3 o'clock positions.

Mirrors

Adjust Rearview and Side Mirrors

• Position your mirrors so that you can see clearly without having to tilt or twist your head excessively.

• Proper mirror adjustment helps maintain good posture by minimising the need for awkward movements.

Take Regular Breaks

Plan Breaks During Long Drives

• During long drives, take breaks every 1-2 hours to get out of the car, stretch, and walk around. This helps relieve pressure on your spine and improves circulation.

• Use the break to reset your posture and make any necessary adjustments to your seat before continuing your journey.

Use Additional Accessories if Needed

Seat Cushions

• If your driving seat is too firm or lacks proper cushioning, consider using an ergonomic seat cushion to improve comfort and support.

Back Support Cushions

• If you need extra support, use a back support cushion to maintain proper spinal alignment during your drive.

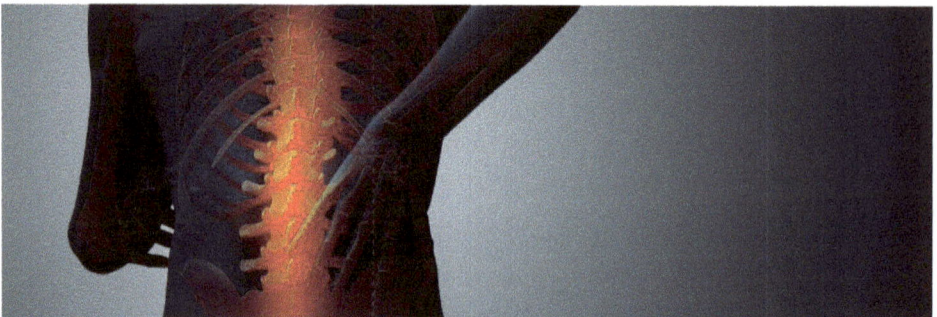

Properly adjusting your seat is crucial for preventing back pain during long drives. By ensuring your seat height, angle, distance, and lumbar support are correctly set, you can reduce strain on your back and maintain a comfortable, supportive posture. Regular breaks, proper headrest positioning, and the use of additional ergonomic accessories can further enhance your comfort and protect your spine during extended periods of driving. If you experience persistent discomfort while driving, consider consulting with a healthcare provider or ergonomic specialist for personalised advice and adjustments.

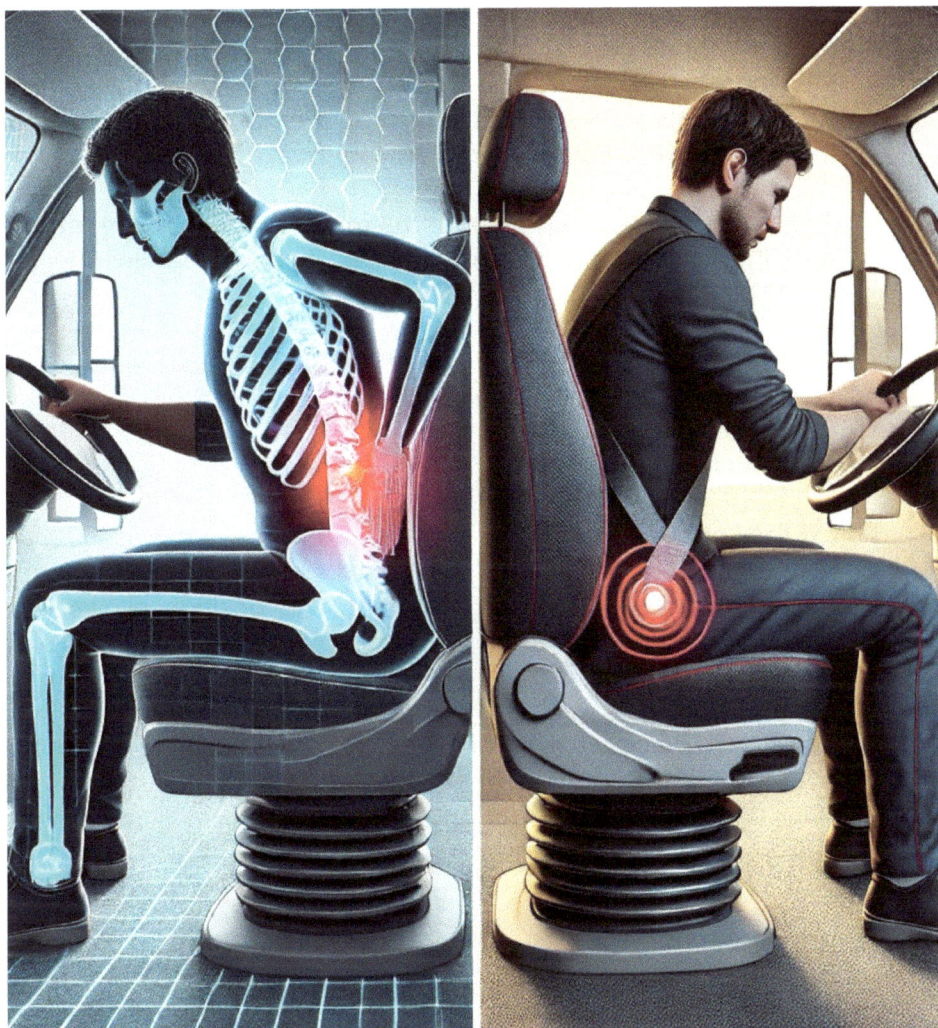

WHAT IS THE OPTIMAL SEAT POSITION AND ANGLE TO REDUCE BACK STRAIN WHILE DRIVING?

Proper seat positioning and angle adjustment are crucial for reducing back strain during driving. The goal is to maintain a neutral spine position, support your lower back, and ensure that your body is aligned correctly to minimise stress on your back and neck. Here's how to achieve the optimal seat position and angle:

Seat Height

- **Adjust the Seat Height:**
  - Position your seat so that your hips are level with or slightly higher than your knees. This helps maintain the natural curve of your lower spine and reduces strain on your back.

  - Ensure you have a clear view of the road and dashboard without needing to stretch or slump. Your head should be close to the ceiling but not touching it.

  - Your feet should comfortably reach the pedals, allowing you to press them fully without stretching your legs.

Seat Distance from Pedals

- **Adjust the Seat Distance:**
  - Slide your seat forward or backward until you can reach the pedals with your knees slightly bent. This position allows your legs to engage the pedals fully without overextending or straining your lower back.

  - You should be able to depress the pedals without having to move your lower back away from the seatback. This ensures that your back remains supported throughout the drive.

Seat Angle

- **Recline the Seatback:**
  - The seatback should be reclined at an angle of about 100 to 110 degrees. This slight recline helps maintain the natural curve of your lumbar spine and reduces the pressure on your lower back.

  - Avoid reclining the seat too far back, as this can cause you to slouch forward, which can strain your neck and upper back.

Lumbar Support

- **Use Built-In Lumbar Support:**
  - If your car seat has adjustable lumbar support, position it to fit the natural curve of your lower back. The support should fill the gap between your lower back and the seatback, providing consistent support during the drive.

  - External Lumbar Cushion: If your car seat doesn't have built-in lumbar support, consider using an external lumbar cushion or roll to maintain proper lower back support.

Seat Cushion Angle (Seat Tilt)

- **Adjust Seat Tilt:**
  - If your seat allows for seat cushion angle adjustment (seat tilt), set it so that your thighs are fully supported without putting pressure on the back of your knees.

  - A slight downward tilt of the seat cushion (toward the back) can help promote a more comfortable and neutral sitting posture, reducing strain on your lower back.

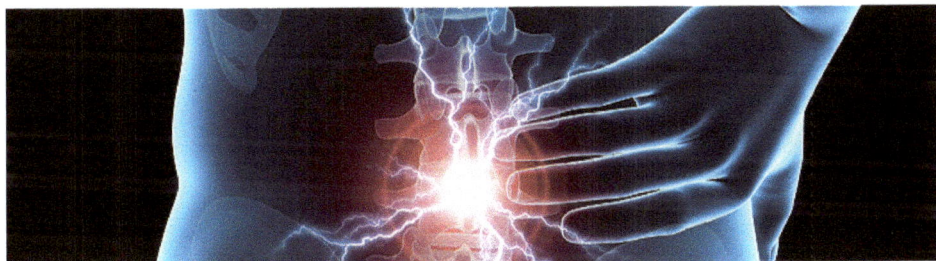

Headrest Position

- **Position the Headrest:**
  - Adjust the headrest so that the top is at least as high as the top of your head, and it's positioned close to the back of your head (within about 2 inches or 5 centimetres). This positioning helps prevent neck strain and whiplash injuries in the event of a collision.

  - The headrest should support the middle of the back of your head to maintain proper alignment with your spine.

Steering Wheel Position

- **Adjust the Steering Wheel:**
  - Position the steering wheel so that you can hold it comfortably with your arms slightly bent at about a 120-degree angle. This reduces strain on your shoulders and upper back.

  - The steering wheel should be close enough that you can reach it without stretching but far enough that there is a gap of about 10-12 inches between your chest and the wheel.

  - Adjust the tilt of the steering wheel so that your hands are in a comfortable position, usually at the 9 and 3 o'clock positions, allowing for easy control without straining your wrists or arms.

Mirrors

- **Adjust Mirrors:**
  - Adjust your rearview and side mirrors to minimise the need for excessive head and neck movement. You should be able to see clearly without twisting your torso.

  - Proper mirror adjustment helps maintain a relaxed and neutral posture while driving, reducing the risk of strain.

Breaks and Movement

- **Take Regular Breaks:**
  - During long drives, take breaks every 1-2 hours to get out of the car, stretch, and walk around. This helps relieve pressure on your spine, improves circulation, and reduces muscle fatigue.

  - Use the break to reset your posture and make any necessary adjustments to your seat before continuing your journey.

The optimal seat position and angle for reducing back strain while driving involve a combination of correct seat height, seatback recline, distance from pedals, and lumbar support. By adjusting these elements to support your natural spinal alignment and promote a neutral posture, you can significantly reduce the risk of back pain and discomfort during long drives. Remember to adjust the headrest and steering wheel to further enhance comfort and safety.

Taking regular breaks and making small adjustments as needed will help keep your body relaxed and comfortable, ensuring a more enjoyable driving experience. If you experience persistent discomfort while driving, then consult an ergonomic specialist if necessary.

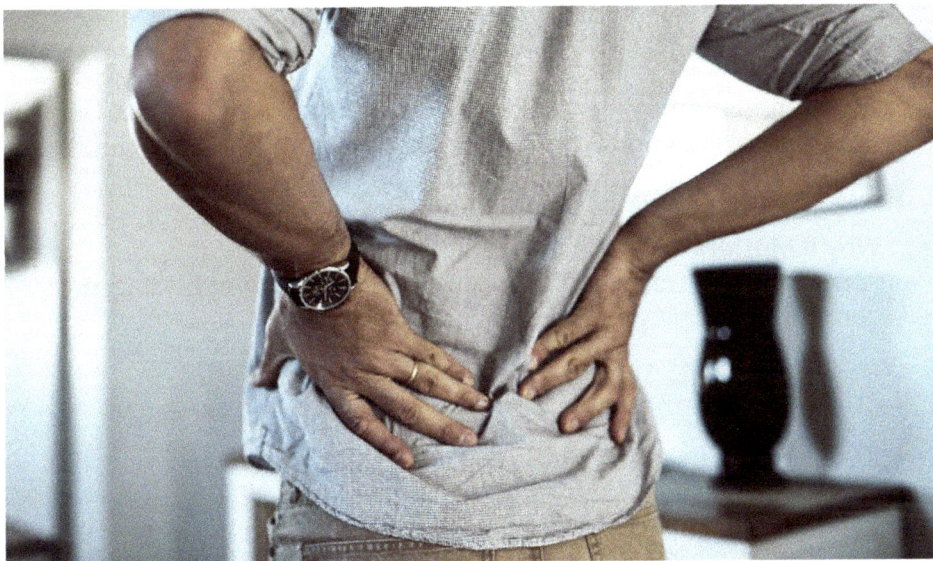

HOW OFTEN SHOULD I TAKE BREAKS TO STRETCH OR WALK AROUND TO PREVENT BACK PAIN DURING LONG TRIPS?

To prevent back pain during long trips, it's important to take regular breaks to stretch and walk around. These breaks help relieve pressure on your spine, improve circulation, and reduce muscle stiffness. Here's a guideline on how often you should take breaks and what you can do during these breaks:

Recommended Frequency for Breaks

Every 1-2 Hours:

- **What to Do:**
  Plan to take a break every 1 to 2 hours of continuous driving. This break should last about 5-10 minutes.

- **Why It Matters:**
  Sitting for extended periods can lead to muscle fatigue, stiffness, and increased pressure on your lower back and spine. Regular breaks help mitigate these effects.

Shorter, More Frequent Breaks:

- **What to Do:**
  If you find yourself experiencing discomfort or stiffness sooner, consider taking shorter, more frequent breaks (every 45 minutes to 1 hour).

- **Why It Matters:**
  Some people may need more frequent breaks depending on their comfort level and any pre-existing back issues.

What to Do During Breaks

Stretching Exercises:

- **Back Stretch:**
  Stand up straight, place your hands on your lower back, and gently arch your back, looking up at the sky. Hold for 10-15 seconds to relieve tension in your lower back.

- **Hamstring Stretch:**
  - Place one foot on a low surface (like a car step or curb) and gently lean forward from your hips, keeping your back straight, to stretch your hamstrings.

  - Hip Flexor Stretch: Step one foot forward into a lunge position, keeping your back leg straight and your front knee bent at 90 degrees. Push your hips forward slightly to stretch your hip flexors.

  - Neck Stretch: Tilt your head towards each shoulder, holding for 15-20 seconds on each side to stretch the neck muscles.

  - Shoulder Rolls: Roll your shoulders backward and forward in a circular motion to relieve tension in your shoulders and upper back.

Walk Around:
- **Short Walk:**
  Take a brisk walk around the rest area, parking lot, or any safe area to get your blood flowing and relieve stiffness in your legs and lower back.

- **Why It Matters:**
  Walking helps to reduce stiffness, improve circulation, and refresh your muscles after sitting for an extended period.

3. **Hydrate and Refresh:**
   - Drink Water: Use the break to drink water and stay hydrated, which is important for overall muscle function and preventing cramps.

   - Light Snack: Consider having a light, healthy snack if needed, to keep your energy levels up, especially on longer trips.

Additional Tips for Long Trips

- **Adjust Your Seat:**
  - Recheck Seat Position: Each time you return to your vehicle, reassess your seat position to ensure it's still providing proper support. Adjust the lumbar support, seat angle, or seat height as needed.

- **Use Supportive Accessories:**
  - Lumbar Support Cushion: Consider using a lumbar support cushion if your car seat doesn't provide adequate lower back support. This can help maintain the natural curve of your spine.

  - Seat Cushions: If your seat is too firm, a cushioned seat pad can help provide additional comfort.

- **Maintain Good Posture:**
  - While Driving: Keep your back straight, shoulders relaxed and avoid slouching. Use both hands on the steering wheel to maintain a balanced posture.

  - Headrest Position: Ensure the headrest is properly adjusted to support your head and neck, reducing strain.

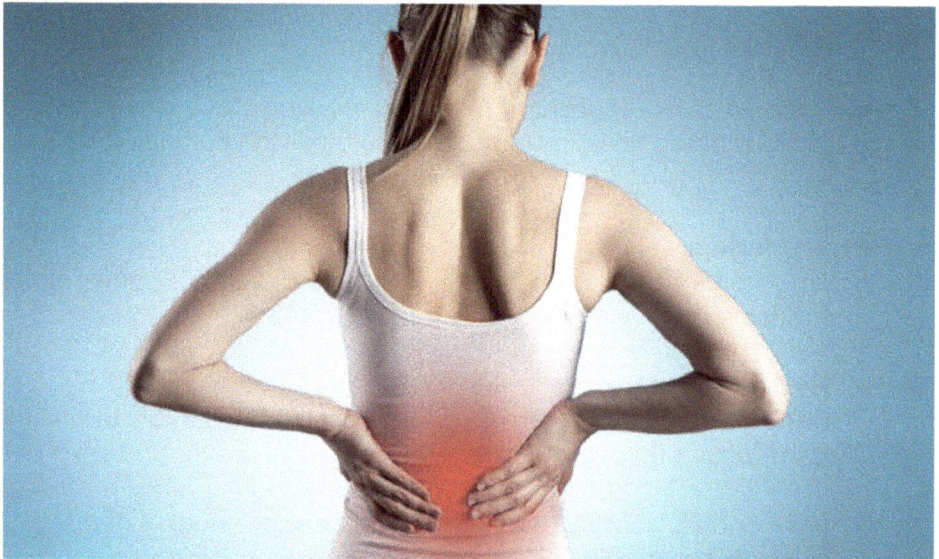

To prevent back pain during long trips, it's important to take breaks every 1 to 2 hours to stretch, walk around, and refresh. During these breaks, perform stretching exercises targeting your back, legs, and neck, and take a short walk to relieve stiffness and improve circulation. Additionally, staying hydrated and adjusting your seat for optimal support will further help in preventing discomfort.

By incorporating these practices into your travel routine, you can reduce the risk of back pain and make your journey more comfortable and enjoyable. If you find that even with regular breaks, you're still experiencing significant discomfort, it may be helpful to consult with a healthcare provider for further investigation or advice.

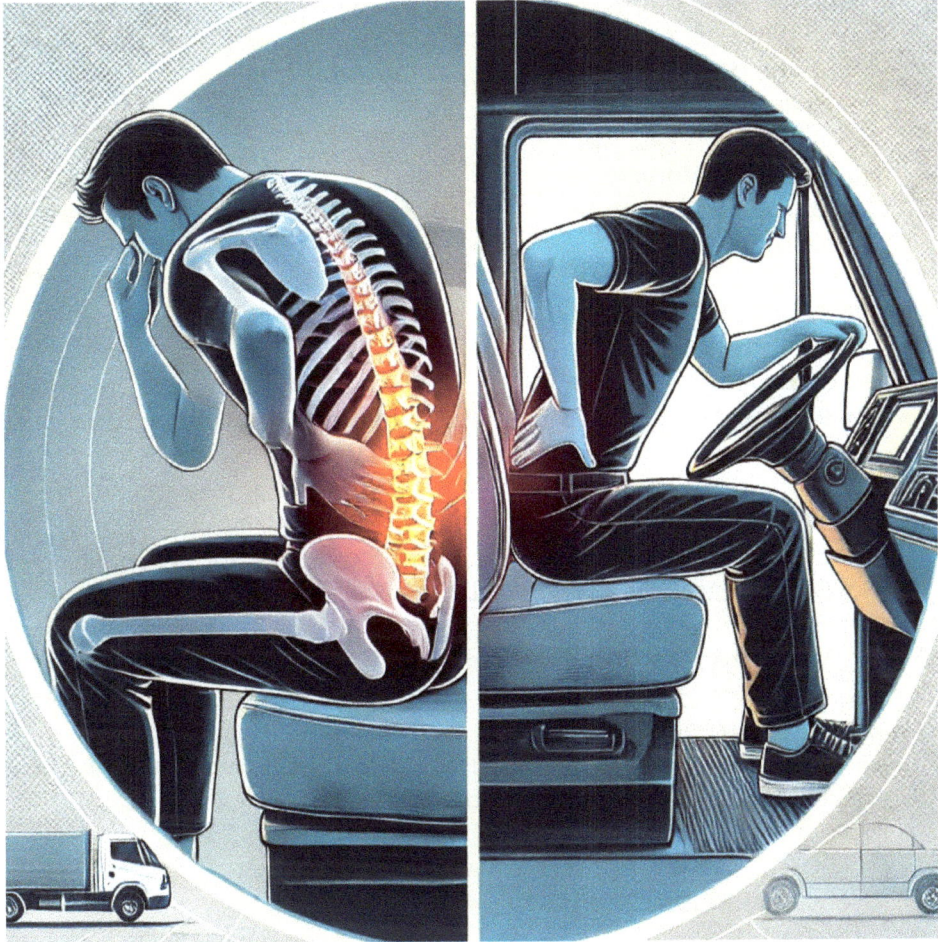

WHAT IS THE BEST WAY TO ENTER AND EXIT MY VEHICLE TO AVOID AGGRAVATING MY BACK PAIN?

Entering and exiting your vehicle correctly can help avoid aggravating back pain by minimising the strain on your back and reducing the risk of awkward movements. Here's a step-by-step guide on the best way to enter and exit your vehicle to protect your back:

Best Way to Enter Your Vehicle

Position Yourself Properly:

- **Stand Close:**
  Stand close to the vehicle, facing away from the door. Your back should be aligned with the seat, and your body should be positioned centrally in front of the seat.

- **Hold onto the Vehicle:**
  Place one hand on the back of the seat or the top of the door frame for support.

Lower Yourself Gently:

- **Backside First:**
  Lower your body into the seat by gently sitting down with your backside first. Avoid bending or twisting your spine.

- **Use Your Legs:**
  Bend your knees and use your leg muscles to lower yourself down slowly and carefully. Keep your back straight as you sit.

Swing Your Legs In:

- **Bring in Your Legs Together:**
  Once seated, pivot on your backside and bring your legs into the vehicle together. This motion should be smooth, avoiding any twisting of your torso.

- **Use Your Hands for Support:**
  If needed, use your hands to help guide your legs or stabilise yourself as you swing them into the car.

Adjust Your Position:

- **Settle into the Seat:**
Once inside, adjust your seating position to ensure your back is properly supported. Use lumbar support or adjust the seat as necessary to maintain good posture.

Best Way to Exit Your Vehicle

Prepare to Exit:
- Reposition Yourself: Before exiting, place your hips and backside to the edge of the seat, facing the door. Ensure your feet are positioned together, ready to swing out of the vehicle.

- Hold onto the Vehicle: Place one hand on the door frame or top of the seat for support.

Swing Your Legs Out:
- Move Legs Together: Pivot on your backside and swing both legs out of the car together. Avoid twisting your torso as you move your legs.

- Keep Your Back Straight: Throughout the movement, keep your back straight to prevent unnecessary strain.

Stand Up Using Your Legs:
- Use Your Legs to Rise: With your legs outside the car and feet firmly planted on the ground, lean forward slightly, and use your leg muscles to push yourself up into a standing position. Avoid using your back muscles to lift yourself up.

- Hold for Support: Use your hands on the door frame, seat, or steering wheel for additional support as you stand.

Avoid Twisting Movements:
- Straight Movements: Throughout the entire process, make sure to keep your movements as straight and controlled as possible. Twisting while getting in or out of the car can aggravate back pain.

Additional Tips for Protecting Your Back

- **Seat Position:**
  Adjust the seat to a higher position, if possible, to make it easier to enter and exit the vehicle without excessive bending.

- **Steady Yourself:**
  If needed, use a walking aid or brace to steady yourself while entering or exiting, particularly if you have significant back pain or mobility issues.

- **Take Your Time:**
  Don't rush the process of getting in or out of the car. Move slowly and deliberately to minimise the risk of straining your back.

By following these steps to enter and exit your vehicle, you can minimise strain on your back and reduce the risk of aggravating back pain. The key is to use your legs for support, avoid twisting your torso, and keep your back as straight as possible during the movements. Taking your time and using your hands for additional support will further help in preventing discomfort and protecting your back health.

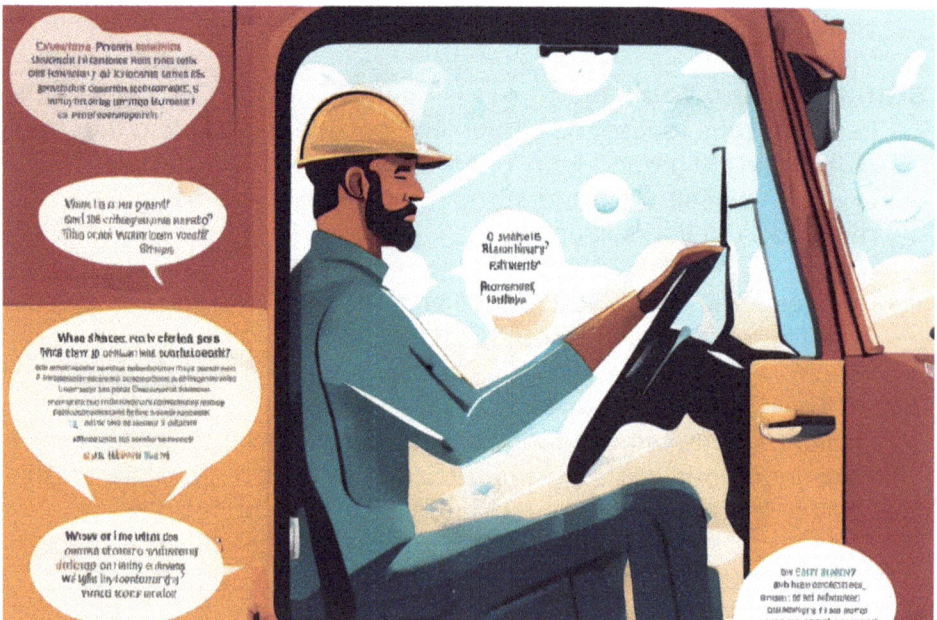

HOW CAN I MODIFY MY STEERING WHEEL POSITION TO MINIMISE BACK DISCOMFORT?

Modifying your steering wheel position can significantly help in minimising back discomfort while driving. The goal is to ensure that the steering wheel is positioned in a way that allows you to maintain a comfortable, relaxed posture without straining your back, shoulders, or arms. Here's how to adjust your steering wheel for optimal comfort:

Adjust the Steering Wheel Height

Position It at Chest Level
- The steering wheel should be adjusted so that it is at or slightly below chest level. This allows your arms to be positioned comfortably at a slight downward angle, reducing strain on your shoulders and upper back.

- Avoid positioning the steering wheel too high, as this can force your shoulders to lift, leading to tension and discomfort.

Adjust the Steering Wheel Distance

Distance from Your Body
- The steering wheel should be close enough that you can reach it without leaning forward, but far enough that there is a gap of about 10-12 inches (25-30 cm) between your chest and the steering wheel. This distance ensures safety in case of airbag deployment and allows you to maintain a relaxed posture.

- Your elbows should be slightly bent (at about a 120-degree angle) when holding the steering wheel, which helps reduce strain on your arms and shoulders.

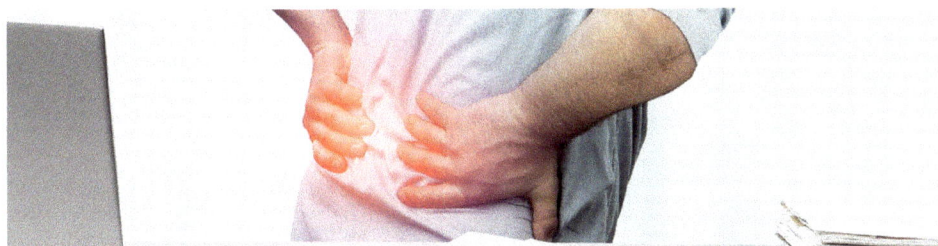

Adjust the Steering Wheel Tilt (Angle)

Tilt to Your Comfort
- Tilt the steering wheel so that your hands naturally fall at the 9 and 3 o'clock positions (or slightly lower at 8 and 4 o'clock). This angle allows your wrists to stay in a neutral position and reduces strain on your arms and back.

- The top of the steering wheel should not obstruct your view of the road or the dashboard. Adjust the tilt to ensure clear visibility while maintaining comfort.

Maintain a Relaxed Grip

Relax Your Grip
- Hold the steering wheel with a relaxed, light grip to reduce muscle tension in your hands, arms, and shoulders. A tight grip can cause unnecessary strain and lead to discomfort over time.

- Consider adjusting your hand position periodically to prevent stiffness and promote circulation.

Use Lumbar Support

Adjust Seat and Lumbar Support
- Before adjusting the steering wheel, ensure that your seat is properly adjusted with adequate lumbar support. Your back should be fully supported by the seat, maintaining the natural curve of your lower spine.

- Sit back in your seat with your back straight and shoulders relaxed. Once your seat is adjusted, modify the steering wheel position to suit your posture.

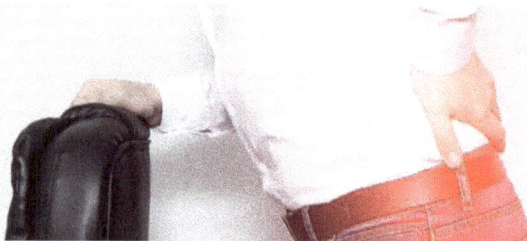

Ensure Proper Posture

Maintain Neutral Spine Alignment

- Keep your back straight and aligned with the seatback. Avoid leaning forward or hunching over the steering wheel, as this can lead to strain on your lower back and neck.

- Your head should be centred and aligned with your spine, and your shoulders should remain relaxed.

Reassess After Adjustments

Test and Adjust

- After adjusting the steering wheel, take a short drive to test the new position. Ensure that you can reach all controls comfortably and that you're not straining any part of your body.

- Make any further adjustments as needed to find the most comfortable and supportive position.

Properly adjusting your steering wheel can significantly reduce back discomfort while driving by promoting good posture and reducing strain on your back, shoulders, and arms. The key is to position the steering wheel at a height and distance that allows you to maintain a relaxed, comfortable posture with slightly bent elbows and a neutral spine. Regularly reassessing your position and adjusting as needed can help you maintain comfort during long drives.

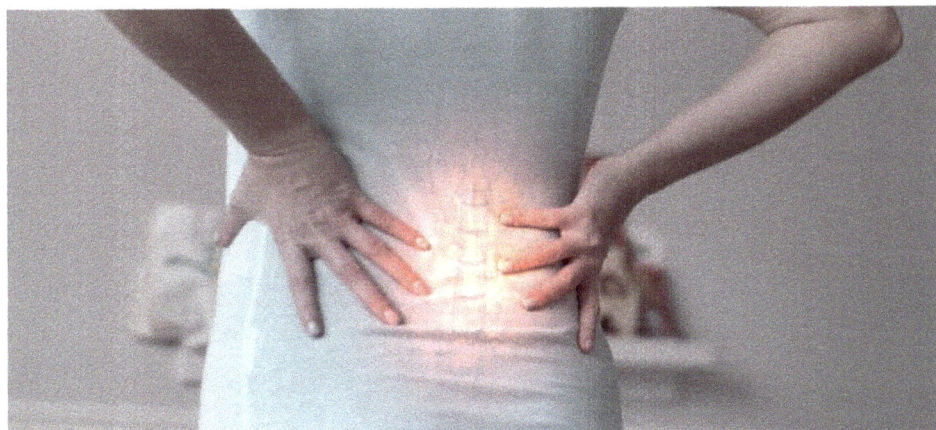

ARE THERE ANY SPECIFIC EXERCISES OR STRETCHES I CAN DO WHILE SITTING IN THE DRIVER'S SEAT TO RELIEVE BACK TENSION?

There are specific exercises and stretches you can do while sitting in the driver's seat to relieve back tension. These exercises can help improve circulation, reduce muscle stiffness, and alleviate discomfort during long drives. Here are some effective stretches and exercises you can perform:

Seated Pelvic Tilts:

How to Do It:
- Sit up straight with your feet flat on the floor and your hands on your thighs.

- Gently tilt your pelvis forward, arching your lower back slightly.

- Then, tilt your pelvis backward, flattening your lower back against the seat.

- Repeat this motion 10-15 times to mobilise your lower back.

Benefits:
- This exercise helps to relieve tension in the lower back and improve flexibility in the spine.

Seated Spinal Twist:

How to Do It:
- Sit up straight with your feet flat on the floor.

- Place your left hand on the outside of your right thigh.

- Gently twist your torso to the right, using your hand to deepen the stretch.

- Hold the stretch for 10-15 seconds, then switch sides.

- Repeat 2-3 times on each side.

Benefits:
* This stretch helps relieve tension in the middle and lower back, as well as the oblique muscles.

Shoulder Shrugs and Rolls:

How to Do It:
* Sit up straight with your hands resting on your lap.

* Shrug your shoulders up towards your ears, hold for a few seconds, then release them down.

* Perform 10 shoulder shrugs.

* Then, roll your shoulders forward in a circular motion 5 times and backward 5 times.

Benefits:
* Shoulder shrugs and rolls help relieve tension in the shoulders and upper back, which can accumulate during long periods of driving.

Neck Stretches:

How to Do It:
* Sit up straight and gently tilt your head to the right, bringing your right ear towards your right shoulder. Hold for 10-15 seconds.

* Repeat on the left side.

* Then, gently tilt your head forward, bringing your chin towards your chest. Hold for 10-15 seconds.

* Finally, gently tilt your head backward, looking up towards the ceiling. Hold for 10-15 seconds.

Benefits:
* These stretches help relieve tension in the neck muscles, which can often become tight during driving.

Seated Cat-Cow Stretch:

How to Do It:
- Sit up straight with your hands on your thighs.

- Inhale and arch your back, bringing your chest forward and lifting your chin slightly (Cat position).

- Exhale and round your back, tucking your chin towards your chest and pulling your belly in (Cow position).

- Repeat this motion 10-15 times.

Benefits:
- This stretch helps mobilise the spine and release tension in the back and shoulders.

Glute Squeeze:

How to Do It:
- Sit up straight with your feet flat on the floor.

- Tighten your glute muscles (buttocks) and hold the contraction for 5-10 seconds, then release.

- Repeat 10-15 times.

Benefits:
- This exercise helps improve circulation in the lower back and glutes, which can reduce stiffness and discomfort during long drives.

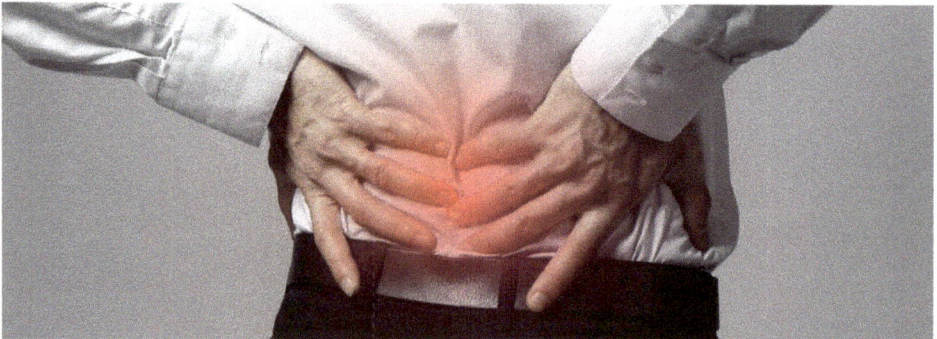

Ankle Pumps:

How to Do It:
- Sit up straight with your feet flat on the floor.

- Lift your heels off the floor while keeping your toes on the ground, then press your heels down and lift your toes off the floor.

- Alternate this movement for 20-30 repetitions.

Benefits:
- Ankle pumps help improve circulation in your legs, reducing the risk of stiffness and swelling.

Tips for Performing These Exercises:

Safety First

Only perform these exercises when the vehicle is stationary, such as during a break or while parked. Never attempt to do these stretches while driving.

Breathe Deeply

Focus on your breathing while performing these stretches. Deep breaths can help enhance relaxation and reduce muscle tension.

Stay Hydrated

Drink water during breaks to stay hydrated, which can help prevent muscle cramps and stiffness.

Incorporating these simple exercises and stretches into your routine during long drives can help relieve back tension and improve your overall comfort. Remember to take regular breaks to get out of the car, stretch your legs, and walk around to further reduce the risk of back pain.

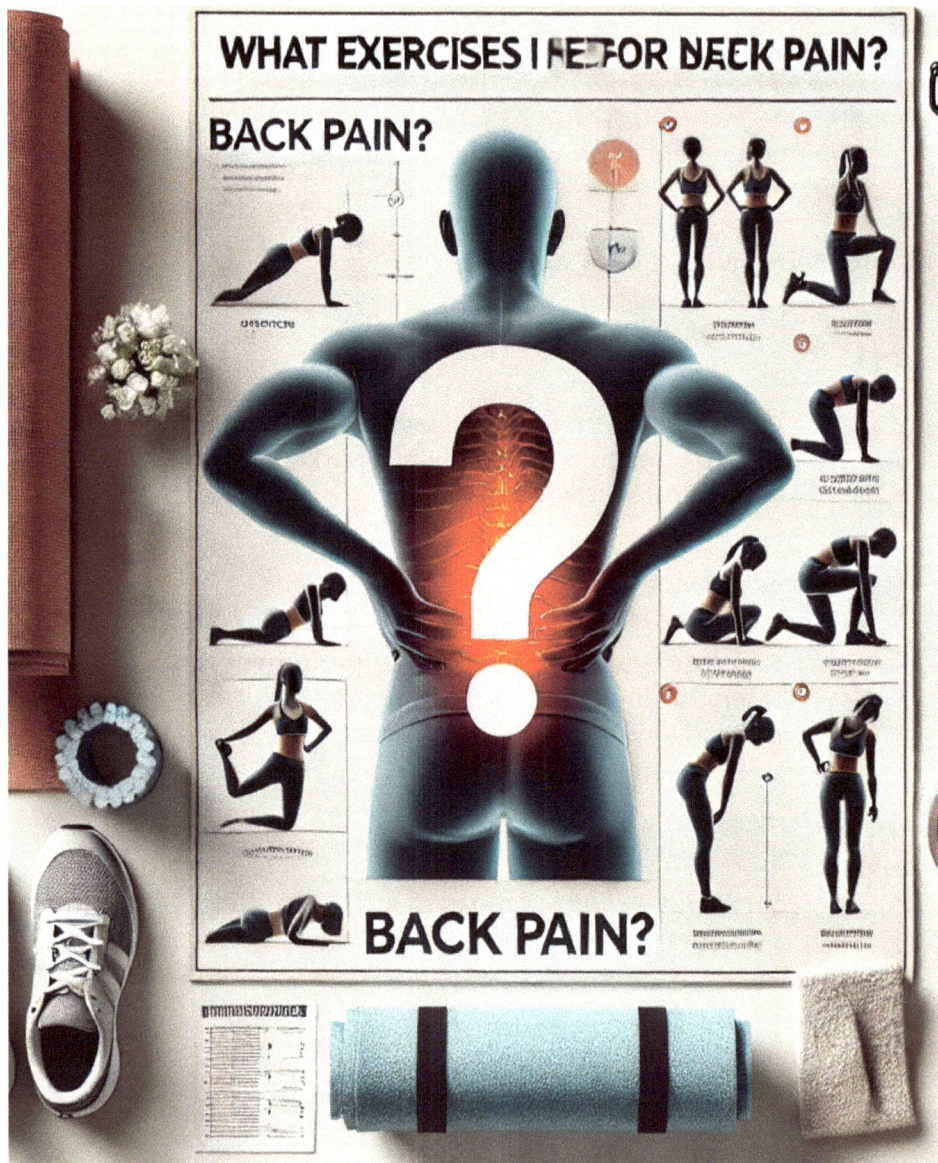

CAN ADJUSTING THE POSITION OF MY MIRRORS REDUCE THE STRAIN ON MY BACK AND NECK?

Yes, adjusting the position of your mirrors can reduce strain on your back and neck by promoting better posture and minimising the need for awkward movements while driving. Properly positioned mirrors help you maintain a more neutral and relaxed posture, reducing the risk of strain and discomfort. Here's how to adjust your mirrors to minimise back and neck strain:

Adjusting the Rearview Mirror

Position for a Straight Posture:
- Sit up straight in your seat, ensuring your back is fully supported by the seatback. Your shoulders should be relaxed, and your head should be in a neutral position, not tilted forward or to the side.

- Adjust the rearview mirror so you can see directly out of the back window without needing to tilt your head or lean forward.

- After adjusting, you should be able to glance at the rearview mirror with just a slight movement of your eyes, not your head. This setup helps maintain proper posture and reduces strain on your neck and upper back.

Adjusting the Side Mirrors

Minimise Head Movement:
- To adjust the side mirrors, sit in your normal driving position. You should be able to see the edge of your vehicle in the mirror without needing to lean or twist your body.

- For the driver's side mirror, lean your head slightly towards the driver's side window and adjust the mirror so that you just see the side of your car. When you return to your normal position, the mirror should give you a wide view of the road beside you.

- For the passenger's side mirror, lean your head towards the centre of the vehicle and adjust the mirror in the same way. This allows you to see more of the road and less of the side of your car, reducing blind spots.

Positioning Tips for Both Mirrors

Field of View:
- Ensure that the mirrors are adjusted to maximise your field of view, covering as much of the road as possible with minimal overlap between the side mirrors and rearview mirror. This setup reduces the need to twist your neck or body to check for traffic in your blind spots.

Mirror Angle:
- Avoid angling the mirrors too far inward or downward, as this can force you to tilt your head or torso to get a clear view. The mirrors should provide a natural view that aligns with your line of sight.

Checking and Adjusting Regularly

Reassess After Seat Adjustments:
- If you adjust your seat position, lumbar support, or steering wheel, reassess your mirror positions to ensure they still align with your new posture.

Regular Adjustments:
- Make a habit of checking your mirror positions periodically, especially after someone else has driven your vehicle or if you notice any discomfort while driving.

Additional Tips to Reduce Strain

- Take Breaks: During long drives, take breaks every 1-2 hours to stretch, walk around, and reset your posture. This helps prevent stiffness and reduces strain on your back and neck.

- Proper Seat Position: Ensure your seat is properly adjusted for comfort and support. Your seatback should be slightly reclined (around 100-110 degrees) to maintain a neutral spine, and your knees should be at the same level or slightly lower than your hips.

- Avoid Overreaching: Keep frequently used items, such as your phone or sunglasses, within easy reach to avoid twisting or stretching your body.

Adjusting the position of your mirrors correctly can play a significant role in reducing strain on your back and neck while driving. By ensuring that your mirrors are aligned with your natural line of sight and require minimal head or body movement to use, you can maintain better posture, minimise discomfort, and drive more comfortably. Regularly checking and adjusting your mirrors, along with proper seat positioning, will further enhance your driving experience and help prevent back and neck strain.

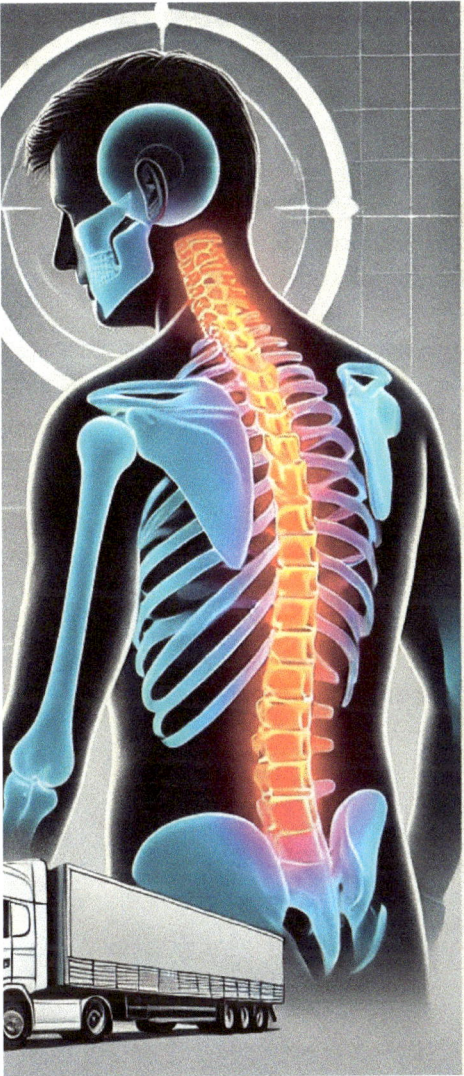

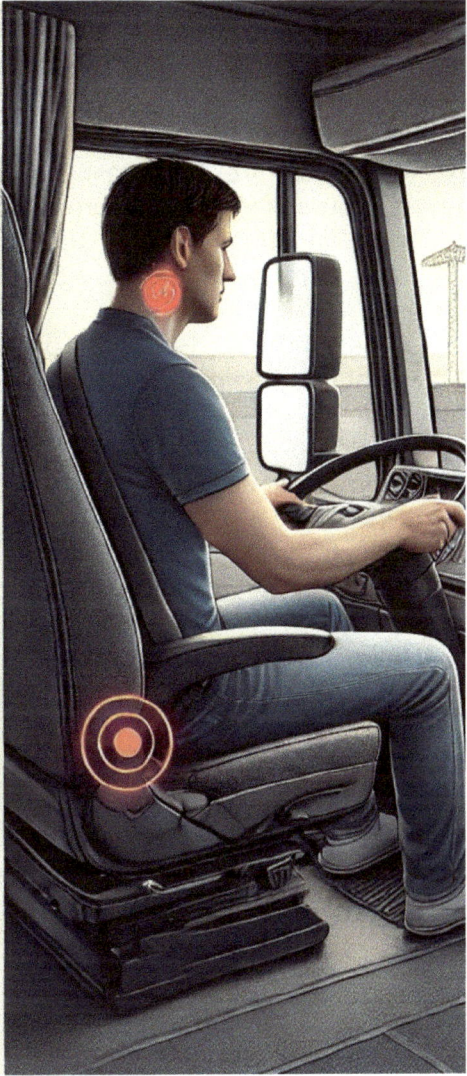

ARE THERE VEHICLE MODIFICATIONS, SUCH AS CUSTOMISED SEATS OR CONTROLS, WHICH COULD HELP MANAGE MY BACK PAIN MORE EFFECTIVELY?

Yes, there are several vehicle modifications, including customised seats and controls, which can help manage back pain more effectively. These modifications are designed to provide better support, improve posture, and reduce strain on your back during driving. Here are some options to consider:

Custom or Ergonomic Car Seats:

Custom-Fit Seats:
- What They Are: Custom-fit seats are designed to match the specific contours of your body, providing personalised support to your back, hips, and thighs. These seats can be particularly beneficial if you have chronic back pain or specific spinal conditions.

- Benefits: Custom-fit seats offer optimal support, reducing pressure points and helping to maintain proper spinal alignment during long drives.

Ergonomic Car Seats:
- What They Are: Ergonomic car seats are designed with features like adjustable lumbar support, memory foam cushioning, and contoured designs that follow the natural curvature of your spine.

- Benefits: These seats can reduce strain on your lower back, improve posture, and provide better overall comfort during driving.

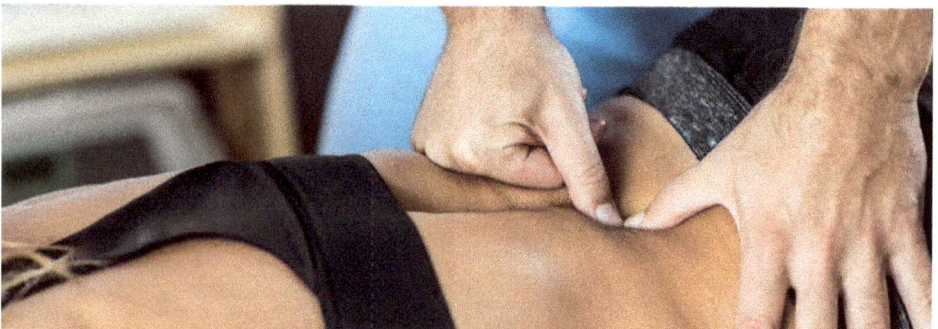

Adjustable Lumbar Support:

Built-In Adjustable Lumbar Support:
- What It Is: Many modern vehicles offer built-in adjustable lumbar support that can be customised to fit the natural curve of your lower back.

- Benefits: Adjusting the lumbar support to your specific needs can help maintain proper spinal alignment and reduce lower back pain, especially on long trips.

Aftermarket Lumbar Cushions:
- What They Are: If your vehicle doesn't have built-in lumbar support, you can add aftermarket lumbar cushions or rolls that provide similar benefits.

- Benefits: These cushions are portable and can be easily adjusted to offer support exactly where you need it.

Heated Seats:

Heated Car Seats:
- What They Are: Heated seats use built-in heating elements to provide warmth to your back and lower body.

- Benefits: Heat therapy can help relax tight muscles, reduce stiffness, and alleviate back pain, making heated seats a valuable feature for managing discomfort during colder weather or long drives.

Aftermarket Lumbar Cushions:
- What They Are: If your vehicle doesn't have built-in lumbar support, you can add aftermarket lumbar cushions or rolls that provide similar benefits.

- Benefits: These cushions are portable and can be easily adjusted to offer support exactly where you need it.

Memory Foam Seat Cushions:

Memory Foam Seat Cushions:

- What They Are: These cushions are made from memory foam, which conforms to your body shape, providing even support and reducing pressure points.

- Benefits: A memory foam cushion can improve comfort by distributing your weight more evenly and reducing strain on your lower back and hips.

Steering Wheel Modifications:

Smaller or Custom Steering Wheels:

- What They Are: A smaller or custom-shaped steering wheel can be easier to manoeuvre, reducing the strain on your shoulders, arms, and back.

- Benefits: These modifications can help you maintain a more comfortable driving posture and reduce fatigue during longer drives.

Steering Wheel Tilt and Telescope Adjustments:

Smaller or Custom Steering Wheels:

- What They Are: Adjustments that allow you to tilt and telescope the steering wheel closer or farther away from you.

- Benefits: These adjustments help you position the steering wheel so that your arms are comfortably bent at the elbows, reducing strain on your back and shoulders.

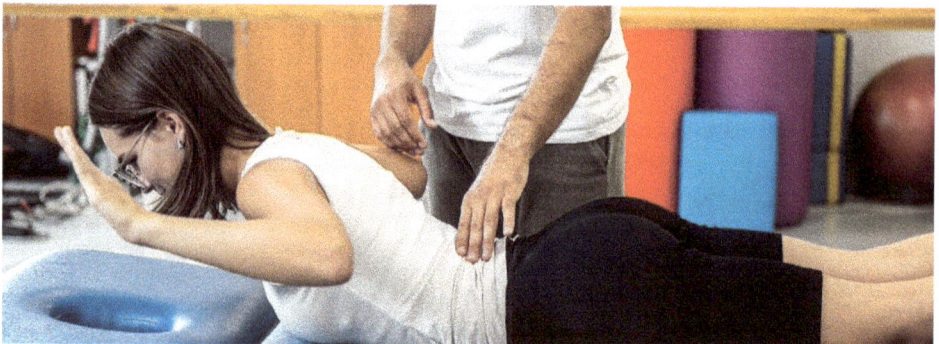

Pedal Extenders:

Pedal Extenders:
- What They Are: Pedal extenders are devices that bring the pedals closer to the driver, which is particularly useful for shorter drivers who may have to stretch their legs to reach the pedals.

- Benefits: By bringing the pedals closer, you can sit with your back fully supported by the seat, reducing strain on your lower back and avoiding overextension of your legs.

Customisable Seat Controls:

Power-Adjustable Seats:
- What They Are: Seats that can be adjusted in multiple ways (height, tilt, recline, lumbar support) using electronic controls.

- Benefits: Power-adjustable seats allow you to find the most comfortable driving position, which can significantly reduce back pain during long drives.

Hand Controls for Acceleration and Braking:

Hand Controls:
- What They Are: Hand controls allow drivers to operate the accelerator and brake pedals using hand-operated levers or buttons, rather than their feet.

- Benefits: This modification can be beneficial for drivers with severe lower back or leg pain, as it reduces the need to press pedals with the feet, which can aggravate back pain.

Suspension Seat:

Suspension Seats:
- What They Are: These seats are designed with built-in suspension systems that absorb shocks and vibrations from the road.

- Benefits: Suspension seats can reduce the impact of bumps and uneven surfaces on your back, making for a smoother and more comfortable ride.

Vehicle Entry and Exit Aids:

Running Boards and Grab Handles:
•   What They Are: Running boards provide a step to make it easier to enter and exit the vehicle, and grab handles offer additional support.

•   Benefits: These aids can help you maintain balance and reduce strain on your back when getting in and out of the car.

Vehicle modifications such as customised seats, adjustable lumbar support, heated seats, and ergonomic steering wheel adjustments can significantly help manage back pain more effectively. These modifications provide better support, reduce strain on your body, and improve overall comfort while driving. Depending on the severity of your back pain and specific needs, you may benefit from one or more of these options. If you experience persistent back pain while driving, consulting with a healthcare provider or an ergonomic specialist can help you determine the best modifications for your situation.

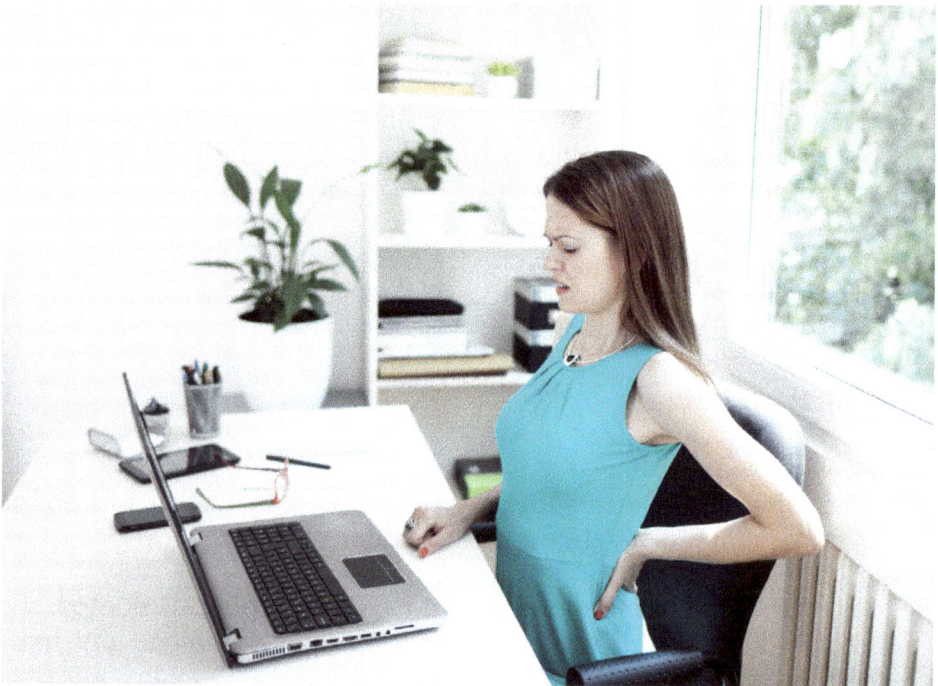

QUESTIONS ABOUT POTENTIAL DIAGNOSTIC TESTS APPLIED FOR BACK PAIN

These questions reflect the concerns that patients often have about the purpose, necessity, and implications of various diagnostic tests related to their back pain.

WHAT TESTS OR SCANS DO I NEED TO DETERMINE THE CAUSE OF MY BACK PAIN?

Determining the cause of back pain often involves a combination of a thorough medical history, physical examination, and diagnostic tests or scans. The specific tests or scans you may need will depend on the nature of your symptoms, their duration, and any other underlying health conditions you might have. Here's an overview of the common diagnostic procedures used to evaluate back pain:

Physical Examination

Purpose: A physical exam allows the doctor to assess your back, posture, and range of motion, and to identify any areas of tenderness, muscle spasms, or neurological deficits (such as weakness, numbness, or reflex changes).

What It Involves: The doctor may ask you to perform certain movements or positions to evaluate pain, flexibility, and nerve function.

X-rays

Purpose: X-rays provide images of the bones in your spine and can help identify structural problems such as fractures, degenerative disc disease, spinal misalignment, or osteoarthritis.

When It's Used: X-rays are typically used as an initial imaging test to rule out fractures, bone abnormalities, or significant spinal deformities.

MRI (Magnetic Resonance Imaging)

Purpose: MRI scans provide detailed images of soft tissues, including discs, muscles, ligaments, nerves, and the spinal cord. They are particularly useful for detecting herniated discs, spinal stenosis, tumours, infections, and nerve root compression.

When It's Used: An MRI is often recommended if you have chronic or severe back pain, neurological symptoms (such as numbness or weakness), or if your doctor suspects a serious underlying condition

CT scan (Computed Tomography)

Purpose: A CT scan provides detailed cross-sectional images of your spine and is often used to evaluate complex bone structures or to get a better look at abnormalities detected on X-rays.

When It's Used: CT scans are often used if MRI is not available or suitable, or to further evaluate abnormalities in the spine, such as spinal stenosis or fractures.

Bone Scans

Purpose: A bone scan can help detect bone abnormalities such as infections, tumours, or fractures that may not be visible on standard X-rays.

When It's Used: Bone scans are typically used when there is a suspicion of bone-related pathology, such as cancer metastasis or osteomyelitis (bone infection).

Electromyography (EMG) and Nerve Conduction Studies

Purpose: EMG measures the electrical activity of muscles, and nerve conduction studies measure how well and how fast the nerves can send electrical signals. These tests can help diagnose nerve compression or damage, such as from a herniated disc or spinal stenosis.

When It's Used: These tests are often used when there are symptoms of nerve involvement, such as numbness, tingling, or muscle weakness, to pinpoint the affected nerves.

Discography

Purpose: Discography involves injecting a contrast dye into the discs of the spine to identify which disc is causing pain. It can help diagnose disc problems when other imaging tests are inconclusive.

When It's Used: Discography is used selectively, often in cases of chronic back pain where the source of pain is unclear, and surgery is being considered.

Ultrasound

Purpose: Ultrasound imaging can be used to evaluate muscles, ligaments, and other soft tissues around the spine. It's less common for diagnosing spinal conditions but can be useful for certain conditions.

When It's Used: Ultrasound is sometimes used to guide injections or in the assessment of soft tissue injuries or abnormalities.

Blood Tests

Purpose: Blood tests can help detect infections, inflammatory conditions (like rheumatoid arthritis), or other systemic conditions that might be causing back pain.

When It's Used: Blood tests are ordered if there is a suspicion of infection, inflammatory arthritis, or other systemic conditions.

Myelography (used rarely if at all)

Purpose: Myelography involves injecting contrast dye into the spinal canal followed by X-rays or CT scans to visualise the spinal cord, nerve roots, and spinal canal.

When It's Used: Myelography is used when MRI is not available or if there is a need for detailed imaging of the spinal canal and nerve roots, especially in cases of spinal stenosis or herniated discs.

Conclusion:

The specific tests or scans you need to determine the cause of your back pain will depend on your symptoms, medical history, and the findings from your physical examination. Your healthcare provider will guide you through the appropriate diagnostic process, which may start with simpler tests like X-rays and progress to more detailed imaging like MRI or CT scans if necessary. If your symptoms are severe, persistent, or associated with neurological deficits, it's important to seek prompt medical evaluation to ensure a proper diagnosis and appropriate treatment plan.

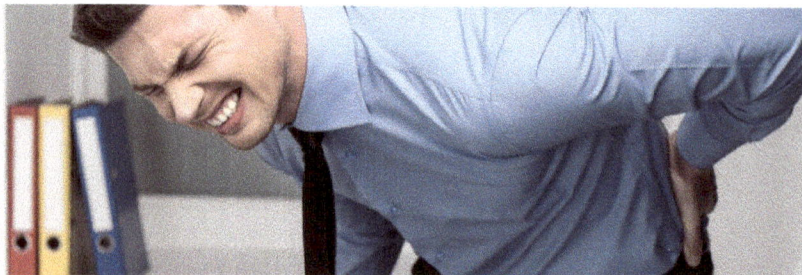

CAN ADJUSTING THE POSITION OF MY MIRRORS REDUCE THE STRAIN ON MY BACK AND NECK?

Yes, adjusting the position of your mirrors can reduce strain on your back and neck by promoting better posture and minimising the need for awkward movements while driving. Properly positioned mirrors help you maintain a more neutral and relaxed posture, reducing the risk of strain and discomfort. Here's how to adjust your mirrors to minimise back and neck strain:

Adjusting the Rearview Mirror

Position for a Straight Posture:
- Sit up straight in your seat, ensuring your back is fully supported by the seatback. Your shoulders should be relaxed, and your head should be in a neutral position, not tilted forward or to the side.

- Adjust the rearview mirror so you can see directly out of the back window without needing to tilt your head or lean forward.

- After adjusting, you should be able to glance at the rearview mirror with just a slight movement of your eyes, not your head. This setup helps maintain proper posture and reduces strain on your neck and upper back.

Adjusting the Side Mirrors

Minimise Head Movement:
- To adjust the side mirrors, sit in your normal driving position. You should be able to see the edge of your vehicle in the mirror without needing to lean or twist your body.

- For the driver's side mirror, lean your head slightly towards the driver's side window and adjust the mirror so that you just see the side of your car. When you return to your normal position, the mirror should give you a wide view of the road beside you.

- For the passenger's side mirror, lean your head towards the centre of the vehicle and adjust the mirror in the same way. This allows you to see more of the road and less of the side of your car, reducing blind spots.

IS AN X-RAY SUFFICIENT TO DIAGNOSE THE CAUSE OF MY BACK PAIN, OR WILL I NEED AN MRI OR CT SCAN?

Whether an X-ray is sufficient to diagnose the cause of your back pain depends on the underlying issue suspected by your healthcare provider. X-rays are a good starting point for diagnosing certain conditions, but they have limitations and may not be enough if your symptoms suggest a more complex or soft tissue-related problem. Here's a breakdown of when an X-ray might be sufficient and when an MRI or CT scan might be necessary:

When an X-ray Might Be Sufficient:

Bone-related Issues:
- Fractures: X-rays are excellent for detecting fractures or broken bones in the spine. If your doctor suspects a vertebral fracture, an X-ray is usually the first imaging test ordered.

- Osteoarthritis: X-rays can reveal signs of osteoarthritis, such as joint space narrowing, bone spurs, or degenerative changes in the spine.

- Spinal Alignment Issues: X-rays are useful for assessing spinal alignment and detecting conditions like scoliosis (abnormal curvature of the spine) or kyphosis (excessive curvature of the upper back).

Initial Assessment:
- Baseline Imaging: X-rays are often used as a first-line diagnostic tool to rule out obvious structural abnormalities in the bones. If the X-ray results are normal, but pain persists, further imaging may be necessary.

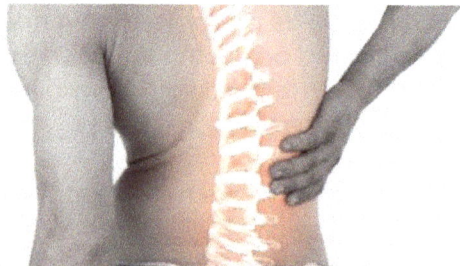

When You Might Need an MRI or CT scan:

Soft Tissue Injuries:

- Herniated Discs: X-rays cannot visualise the discs between the vertebrae. If a herniated or bulging disc is suspected, an MRI is typically required because it provides detailed images of soft tissues.

- Muscle and Ligament Injuries: MRI is also preferred for assessing injuries to the muscles, ligaments, and tendons in the back.

Nerve-related Issues:

- Nerve Compression: If you have symptoms of nerve compression, such as radiating pain, numbness, tingling, or weakness in your legs, an MRI is often needed to evaluate the spinal cord and nerve roots.

- Spinal Stenosis: MRI is the best imaging modality to diagnose spinal stenosis, a condition where the spinal canal narrows and compresses the nerves.

Complex Bone Conditions:

- Spinal Fractures: While X-rays can detect fractures, a CT scan may be needed for a more detailed evaluation, especially if the fracture is complex or involves the spinal cord.

- Bone Tumours or Infections: If there is a suspicion of bone tumours, infections, or other bone abnormalities, a CT scan or MRI may be necessary to get a more comprehensive view.

Persistent or Unexplained Symptoms:

- Chronic Pain: If your back pain is chronic and has not improved with initial treatment, an MRI may be ordered to explore other possible causes that X-rays cannot reveal.

- Inconclusive X-ray Results: If your X-ray is inconclusive but you continue to have significant pain or neurological symptoms, an MRI or CT scan may be required to provide more detailed information.

In summary:

- X-rays are sufficient for diagnosing certain bone-related conditions, such as fractures, osteoarthritis, and spinal alignment issues. They are often the first imaging test used because they are quick, widely available, and cost-effective.

- MRI or CT scans are necessary when the suspected cause of your back pain involves soft tissues (such as discs, muscles, or nerves), when there is a need for detailed imaging of complex bone conditions, or when X-rays do not provide sufficient information.

The choice of imaging depends on your specific symptoms, medical history, and the findings from your physical examination. Your healthcare provider will recommend the most appropriate imaging based on your condition. If you're experiencing symptoms like radiating pain, numbness, or weakness, or if your pain is severe and persistent, an MRI or CT scan may be necessary for a more accurate diagnosis.

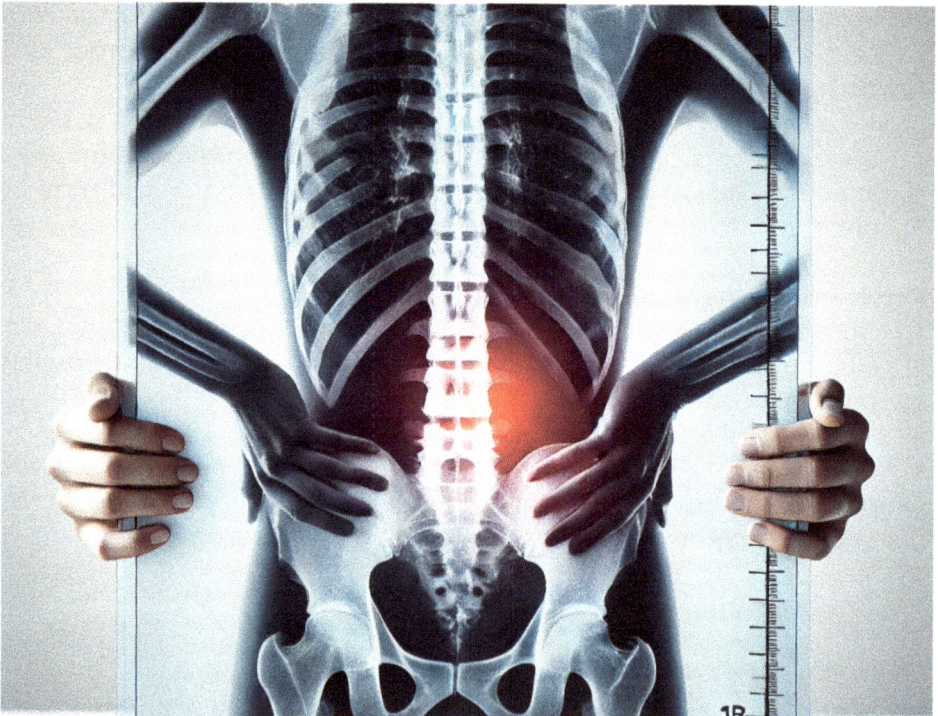

WHAT CAN AN MRI TELL ME ABOUT MY BACK PAIN THAT OTHER TESTS CANNOT?

An MRI (Magnetic Resonance Imaging) is a powerful diagnostic tool that provides detailed images of the soft tissues in your body, including muscles, discs, ligaments, nerves, and the spinal cord. This capability allows an MRI to reveal specific causes of back pain that other imaging tests, like X-rays or CT scans, might miss. Here is what an MRI can tell you about your back pain:

Detailed Imaging of Soft Tissues

Intervertebral Discs:
- What It Shows: MRI can provide detailed images of the intervertebral discs, which are the cushions between the vertebrae. It can detect conditions like herniated discs, bulging discs, and degenerative disc disease.

- Why It Matters: Disc issues are a common cause of back pain, especially if the disc is pressing on nearby nerves.

Spinal Cord and Nerve Roots:
- What It Shows: MRI can visualise the spinal cord and the nerve roots as they exit the spine. It can reveal nerve compression or irritation, which might not be visible on X-rays or CT scans.

- Why It Matters: Nerve-related issues, such as sciatica, are often due to conditions like herniated discs or spinal stenosis, which MRI can clearly show.

Ligaments and Muscles:
- What It Shows: MRI can assess the ligaments and muscles that support the spine, identifying tears, strains, or inflammation.

- Why It Matters: Soft tissue injuries, which might not be evident on other imaging tests, can be a significant source of back pain.

Assessment of Spinal Canal and Nerve Compression

Spinal Stenosis:
- What It Shows: MRI is the gold standard for diagnosing spinal stenosis, which is the narrowing of the spinal canal that can compress the spinal cord or nerves.

- Why It Matters: Spinal stenosis can lead to significant pain, numbness, and weakness, particularly in the legs. MRI can show the extent and location of the narrowing.

Nerve Root Compression:
- What It Shows: MRI can detect nerve root compression, which may be caused by herniated discs, bone spurs, or other spinal abnormalities.

- Why It Matters: Identifying the specific nerve root affected can help tailor treatment plans, such as targeted physical therapy, injections, or surgery.

Evaluation of Bone Marrow and Vertebrae

Bone Marrow Abnormalities:
- What It Shows: MRI can detect abnormalities in the bone marrow, such as tumours, infections, or inflammation.

- Why It Matters: Conditions like metastatic cancer, bone infections, or certain types of arthritis can cause back pain and might only be detected through MRI.

Vertebral Body Issues:
- What It Shows: While CT scans are often used for detailed bone imaging, MRI can still provide valuable information about the condition of the vertebrae, especially when soft tissue involvement is suspected.

- Why It Matters: MRI can help diagnose conditions like vertebral fractures, particularly when associated with bone oedema or other soft tissue changes.

Detection of Inflammatory or Infectious Conditions

Spinal Infections:
- What It Shows: MRI is highly effective at detecting infections in the spine, such as discitis (infection of the intervertebral disc) or osteomyelitis (infection of the bone).

- Why It Matters: Spinal infections are serious and require prompt treatment. MRI is often the best tool for early and accurate diagnosis.

Inflammatory Conditions:
- What It Shows: MRI can show signs of inflammation in the joints of the spine (such as in spondylarthritis) or in the surrounding soft tissues.

- Why It Matters: Early detection of inflammatory conditions can lead to more effective treatment and better outcomes.

Identification of Tumours or Other Masses

Spinal Tumours:
- What It Shows: MRI can detect tumours or abnormal growths in or around the spine, including those affecting the vertebrae, spinal cord, or nerve roots.

- Why It Matters: Identifying tumours is critical for appropriate management, whether through surgery, radiation, or other treatments.

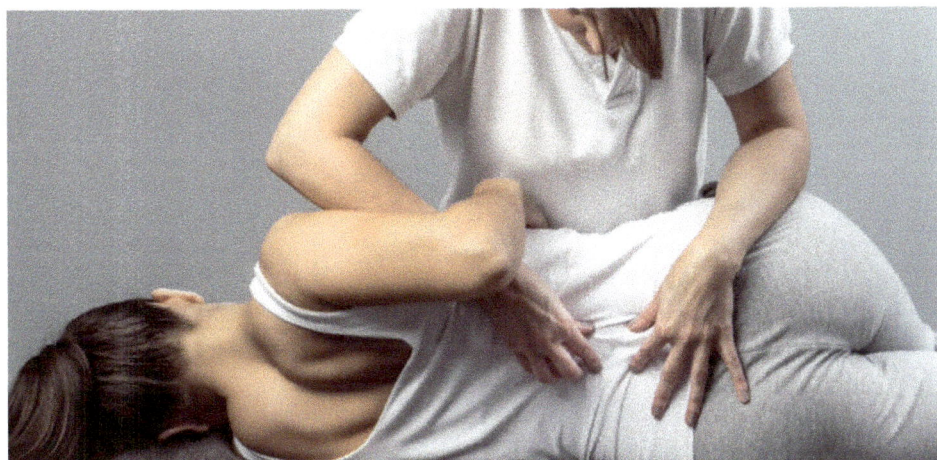

Guidance for Treatment Planning

Precision in Treatment:
- What It Shows: The detailed information provided by an MRI can help in planning treatments, such as targeted physical therapy, epidural steroid injections, or surgical interventions.

- Why It Matters: Accurate diagnosis leads to more effective treatment, potentially preventing the progression of the condition and improving quality of life.

An MRI can provide comprehensive and detailed information about your back pain by visualising soft tissues, nerve structures, and any potential abnormalities that other imaging tests cannot detect. It is particularly valuable for diagnosing conditions like herniated discs, spinal stenosis, nerve compression, spinal infections, and tumours. If your back pain is persistent, severe, or associated with neurological symptoms, an MRI can be an essential tool in identifying the underlying cause and guiding appropriate treatment.

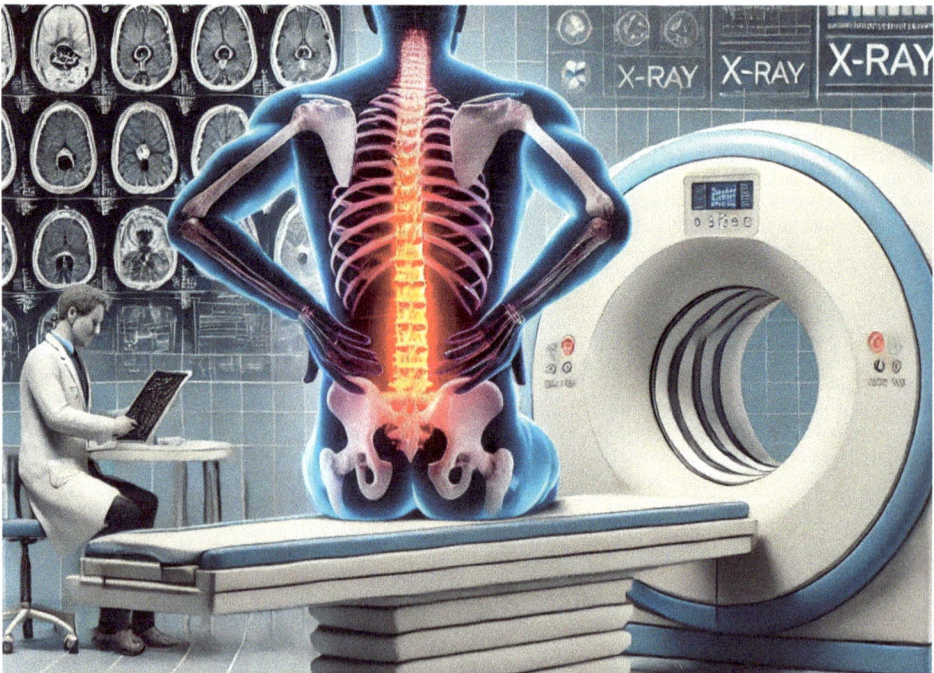

ARE THERE ANY RISKS ASSOCIATED WITH GETTING AN MRI OR CT SCAN FOR MY BACK PAIN?

The easy answer is "no." Both MRI (Magnetic Resonance Imaging) and CT (Computed Tomography) scans are commonly used diagnostic tools that can provide detailed images to help diagnose the cause of back pain. While they are safe, each imaging technique carries certain risks and considerations. Here is an overview of the potential risks associated with each:

Risks Associated with MRI

Magnetic Field Exposure:
- What It Is: MRI uses a strong magnetic field and radio waves to create detailed images of the body.

Risks:
- Metal Implants: The magnetic field can interfere with metal implants such as pacemakers, cochlear implants, or certain types of aneurysm clips. Patients with these implants may be at risk and should discuss their specific situation with their doctor.

- Metal Fragments: If you have any metal fragments in your body, particularly in the eyes, you should inform the healthcare provider as MRI could cause movement or heating of the metal.

Claustrophobia and Discomfort:
- What It Is: MRI scans are performed in a narrow, enclosed tube, which can cause discomfort or anxiety for people with claustrophobia.

Risks:
- Claustrophobia: Some patients may experience significant anxiety or panic while inside the MRI machine. Open MRI machines or sedatives can sometimes be used to alleviate this issue.

- Loud Noise: MRI machines are noisy, which can be uncomfortable. Patients are usually given earplugs or headphones to reduce the noise.

Contrast Agents:
- What It Is: In some cases, a contrast agent (usually gadolinium) is injected into a vein to enhance the images.

Risks:
- Allergic Reactions: Although rare, some people may have an allergic reaction to the contrast agent.

- Kidney Function: In patients with pre-existing kidney problems, there is a risk of a condition called nephrogenic systemic fibrosis (NSF), which is associated with gadolinium-based contrast agents.

Risks Associated with CT scans

Radiation Exposure:
- What It Is: CT scans use X-rays to create detailed cross-sectional images of the body.

Risks:
- Increased Cancer Risk: CT scans expose you to a higher dose of radiation compared to standard X-rays. While the risk is low, repeated exposure to radiation over time can increase the risk of developing cancer.

- Cumulative Exposure: For patients who require multiple CT scans, the cumulative radiation dose can be a concern, particularly for younger patients or those who are otherwise healthy.

Contrast Agents:
- What It Is: Like MRI, CT scans sometimes use contrast agents (usually iodine-based) to enhance the visibility of certain structures.

Risks:
- Allergic Reactions: Iodine-based contrast agents can cause allergic reactions, ranging from mild to severe.

- Kidney Function: Iodine-based contrast can also affect kidney function, especially in patients with pre-existing kidney disease

Potential for False Positives:
- What It Is: CT scans can sometimes reveal abnormalities that are not clinically significant.

Risks:
- Unnecessary Anxiety or Procedures: Discovering incidental findings can lead to further testing or procedures that may not have been necessary, potentially causing unnecessary stress or exposure to additional risks.

Special Considerations:
- Pregnancy: Both MRI and CT scans are avoided during pregnancy unless necessary. MRI is considered safer than CT during pregnancy because it doesn't involve ionising radiation, but it's still used with caution.

- Paediatric Considerations: For children, minimising radiation exposure is a priority, so MRI may be preferred over CT, when possible, although it depends on the clinical situation.

Weighing the Risks and Benefits
While there are risks associated with MRI and CT scans, these risks are outweighed by the benefits of obtaining a clear diagnosis, especially in cases where serious conditions like tumours, infections, or severe structural problems are suspected.

Before undergoing an MRI or CT scan, it's important to discuss your medical history, current medications, and any implants or allergies with your healthcare provider. They can help determine which imaging modality is most appropriate for your situation and how to mitigate any potential risks.

Conclusion
MRI and CT scans are valuable tools for diagnosing back pain, each with its own set of risks and benefits. MRI is safer for soft tissue imaging and doesn't involve radiation, but it can pose risks for people with certain implants or metal fragments. CT scans, while quick and effective for imaging bones and complex structures, do expose patients to ionising radiation, which carries a small risk of cancer with repeated exposure. Your healthcare provider will help you make an informed decision about which test is most appropriate based on your specific symptoms and medical history.

HOW ACCURATE ARE THESE IMAGING TESTS IN IDENTIFYING THE SOURCE OF BACK PAIN?

Imaging tests like X-rays, MRI (Magnetic Resonance Imaging), and CT (Computed Tomography) scans are valuable tools in diagnosing the source of back pain. However, their accuracy in identifying the exact cause of back pain varies depending on the underlying condition and the specific test used. Here's an overview of the accuracy and limitations of these imaging tests:

X-rays:

Accuracy:
- Good for Bone Abnormalities: X-rays are quite accurate for detecting bone-related issues such as fractures, osteoarthritis, spinal alignment issues (like scoliosis), and bone spurs. They can clearly show changes in bone structure and joint space narrowing associated with degenerative conditions.

- Limited for Soft Tissues: X-rays do not provide clear images of soft tissues, such as muscles, ligaments, discs, and nerves. Therefore, they are not effective in diagnosing soft tissue-related causes of back pain, such as herniated discs or muscle strains.

Limitations:
- Cannot Detect Soft Tissue Issues: Because X-rays cannot visualise soft tissues, they may miss the most common sources of back pain, such as disc herniation, nerve compression, or muscle injuries.

- Potential for Overdiagnosis: X-rays may reveal incidental findings like minor osteoarthritis or disc degeneration that might not actually be the cause of pain, leading to potential overdiagnosis.

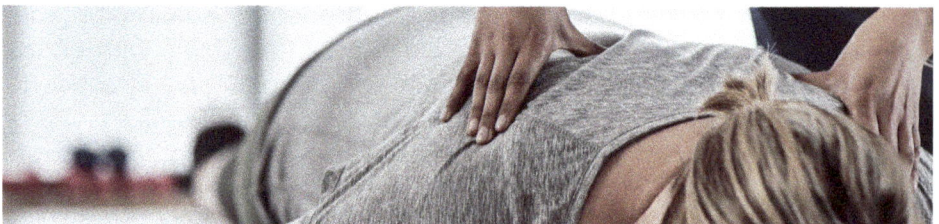

MRI (Magnetic Resonance Imaging)

Accuracy:
- High Accuracy for Soft Tissue Problems: MRI is extremely accurate in detecting soft tissue issues, such as herniated discs, bulging discs, spinal stenosis, ligament or muscle injuries, and nerve root compression. It provides detailed images of the spinal cord, nerves, and discs, making it the preferred test for evaluating complex or unexplained back pain.

- Effective for Identifying Inflammatory or Infectious Conditions: MRI is also highly effective in identifying conditions like spinal infections, tumours, and inflammatory diseases, which can be sources of back pain.

Limitations:
- Incidental Findings: MRI may reveal abnormalities that are not causing symptoms, such as mild disc bulges or degenerative changes that are common in the aging population. These incidental findings can sometimes lead to unnecessary worry or further testing.

- Variability in Interpretation: The interpretation of MRI results can vary among radiologists, and not all findings are clinically significant. It's important for the imaging results to be correlated with clinical symptoms by a knowledgeable healthcare provider.

CT (Computed Tomography) Scan

Accuracy:
- High Accuracy for Bone and Complex Structures: CT scans are very accurate for assessing bone structures, including detecting fractures, bone tumours, and complex spinal abnormalities. They provide detailed cross-sectional images that are particularly useful in evaluating the bony anatomy of the spine.

- Moderate for Soft Tissues: While CT scans can visualise some soft tissue structures, such as discs and spinal canal, they are not as detailed as MRI for soft tissue evaluation.

Limitations:
- Radiation Exposure: CT scans involve exposure to ionising radiation, which is a consideration, especially if multiple scans are needed.

- Less Effective for Detailed Soft Tissue Imaging: Compared to MRI, CT scans are less effective in detecting subtle soft tissue abnormalities, such as small disc herniations or early-stage nerve compression

Ultrasound

Accuracy:
- High Accuracy for Bone and Complex Structures: CT scans are o Limited Use for Back Pain: Ultrasound is not used as a primary imaging modality for back pain. It can be useful for assessing superficial soft tissue injuries or guiding injections but is not effective for evaluating deep structures like the spine and spinal cord.

Limitations:
- Limited Depth and Resolution: Ultrasound lacks the depth and resolution to effectively visualise spinal structures and diagnose most causes of back pain.

Clinical Correlation

Importance of Correlating Imaging with Symptoms:
- Imaging tests should always be interpreted in the context of a patient's clinical history and physical examination. For example, an MRI might show a herniated disc, but if the patient's symptoms don't align with the location of the herniation, it may not be the true source of pain.

- Clinical judgment is essential to determine whether the findings on an imaging test are relevant to the patient's symptoms or if they are incidental.

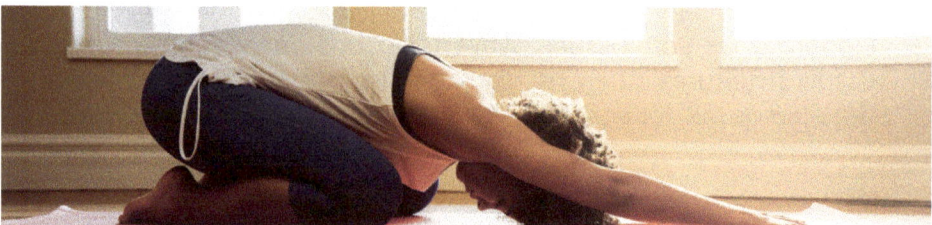

Summarising all the above

- X-rays are accurate for detecting bone-related issues but are limited in evaluating soft tissue problems, which are often the source of back pain.

- MRI is highly accurate for diagnosing soft tissue and nerve-related causes of back pain, such as herniated discs, spinal stenosis, and nerve compression. However, it can also reveal incidental findings that may not be clinically significant.

- CT scans are excellent for detailed imaging of bones and complex structures but are less effective than MRI for soft tissue evaluation. They involve radiation exposure, which is a consideration.

- Ultrasound is not commonly used for diagnosing back pain due to its limitations in visualising deep structures.

Overall, the accuracy of these imaging tests depends on the specific condition being investigated, and they should be used in conjunction with a thorough clinical evaluation. Your healthcare provider will determine the most appropriate imaging test based on your symptoms, medical history, and physical examination findings.

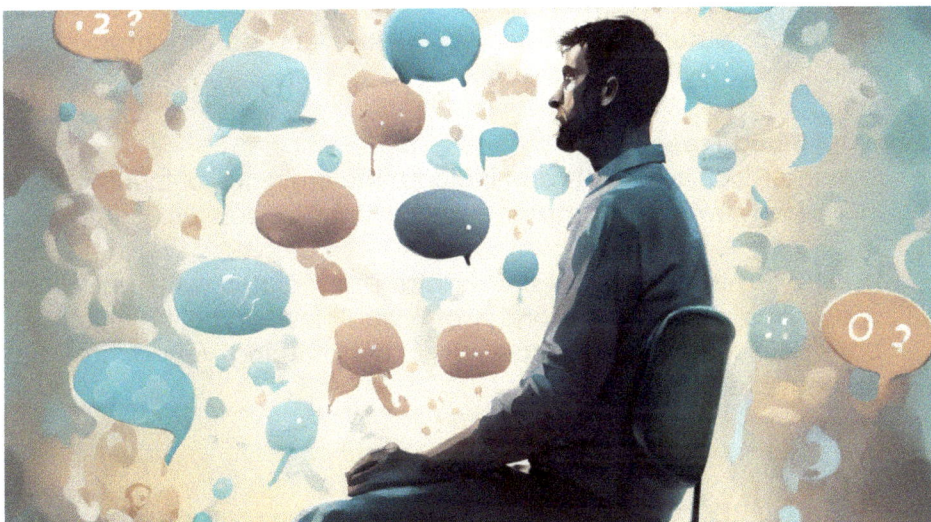

WILL I NEED BLOOD TESTS TO RULE OUT ANY UNDERLYING CONDITIONS CONTRIBUTING TO MY BACK PAIN?

Blood tests are not routinely used to diagnose the cause of back pain, but they can be helpful in certain situations to rule out underlying conditions that might be contributing to your symptoms. Whether you need blood tests depends on the nature of your back pain, your medical history, and the findings from your physical examination. Here are some scenarios where blood tests might be recommended:

Infection
- Why It's Important: Back pain can sometimes be caused by infections such as discitis (infection of the intervertebral discs), osteomyelitis (infection of the bones), or spinal abscesses.

Relevant Blood Tests:
- Complete Blood Count (CBC): A CBC can help identify signs of infection or inflammation, such as an elevated white blood cell count.

- Erythrocyte Sedimentation Rate (ESR) and C-Reactive Protein (CRP): These are markers of inflammation that may be elevated in cases of infection or inflammatory conditions.

Inflammatory or Autoimmune Conditions
- Why It's Important: Conditions like ankylosing spondylitis, rheumatoid arthritis, or other inflammatory conditions can cause chronic back pain, especially in younger adults.

Relevant Blood Tests:
- ESR and CRP: These tests can indicate the presence of inflammation in the body, which is common in autoimmune diseases.

- HLA-B27: This genetic marker is often associated with ankylosing spondylitis and other spondyloarthropathies. If you have chronic back pain with stiffness, especially in the morning, your doctor may order this test.

Cancer or Malignancy

- Why It's Important: Although rare, back pain can sometimes be a symptom of metastatic cancer, particularly in older adults or those with a history of cancer.

Relevant Blood Tests:

- Tumour Markers: Specific markers can be tested if there's a suspicion of certain cancers, though these are not routine for most back pain cases.

- Alkaline Phosphatase: This enzyme can be elevated in bone metastasis or other bone conditions.

- Calcium and Phosphate Levels: Abnormal levels can indicate bone involvement, due to malignancy.

Osteoporosis and Bone Health

- Why It's Important: Osteoporosis can lead to fractures in the spine, which can cause back pain. It's more common in older adults, particularly postmenopausal women.

Relevant Blood Tests:

- Calcium and Vitamin D Levels: Low levels can indicate poor bone health and a risk for osteoporosis.

- Parathyroid Hormone (PTH): Abnormal levels can affect calcium metabolism and bone health.

Kidney Function

- Why It's Important: Back pain can sometimes be related to kidney issues, such as kidney stones or infections, especially if the pain is localised to the lower back or flank area.

Relevant Blood Tests:

- Blood Urea Nitrogen (BUN) and Creatinine: These tests assess kidney function and can indicate whether kidney issues might be contributing to your back pain.

General Inflammatory Markers

- Why It's Important: If your back pain is accompanied by systemic symptoms like unexplained weight loss, fever, or general malaise, blood tests can help determine if there is an underlying inflammatory or systemic condition.

Relevant Blood Tests:

- ESR and CRP: As mentioned earlier, these tests are general markers of inflammation and can point toward an underlying inflammatory or infectious process.

Thyroid Function

- Why It's Important: In some cases, thyroid disorders can contribute to musculoskeletal pain, including back pain.

Relevant Blood Tests:

- Thyroid Function Tests (TSH, Free T4, and Free T3): These tests evaluate thyroid function, which can influence muscle and bone health.

When Blood Tests May Not Be Needed

- Mechanical Back Pain: For most cases of mechanical back pain (e.g., due to muscle strain, herniated discs, or spinal stenosis), blood tests are not typically necessary.

- Acute Injury: If the back pain is clearly related to a specific injury or mechanical cause, imaging tests like X-rays or MRI are usually more appropriate than blood tests.

Blood tests can be an important part of the diagnostic process in certain cases of back pain, particularly when there is a suspicion of an infection, inflammatory condition, malignancy, or other systemic issue. However, they are not routinely required for all patients with back pain. Your healthcare provider will determine whether blood tests are necessary based on your symptoms, medical history, and physical examination findings. If blood tests are indicated, they can provide valuable information to guide further investigation and treatment.

QUESTIONS ABOUT THE WAY DIET IS INFLUENCING BACK PAIN

These questions reflect the common concerns and considerations that back pain sufferers have about how their diet can affect their condition and overall spine health.

ARE THERE SPECIFIC FOODS THAT CAN HELP REDUCE INFLAMMATION AND ALLEVIATE MY BACK PAIN?

Certain foods have anti-inflammatory properties that can help reduce inflammation and may alleviate back pain. Incorporating these foods into your diet can support your overall health and potentially reduce the severity of your back pain. Here's a list of foods that can help reduce inflammation:

Fatty Fish

- Examples: Salmon, mackerel, sardines, trout, and tuna.

- Why They Help: Fatty fish are rich in omega-3 fatty acids, which are known for their strong anti-inflammatory effects. Omega-3s can help reduce inflammation that may contribute to chronic back pain.

- How to Include Them: Aim to include fatty fish in your diet at least two to three times a week. You can grill, bake, or steam them for a healthy meal.

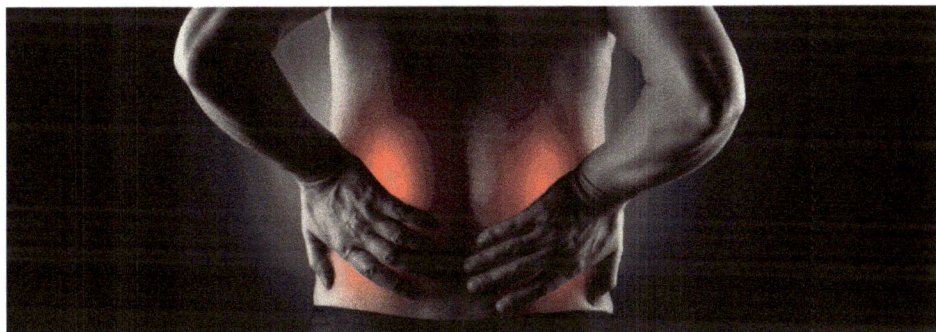

Fruits

- Examples: Berries (strawberries, blueberries, raspberries), cherries, oranges, and pineapples.

- Why They Help: These fruits are high in antioxidants, vitamins, and fibre. Berries and cherries contain anthocyanins, which have been shown to reduce inflammation.

- How to Include Them: Enjoy berries and cherries as snacks, add them to your breakfast cereal or yogurt, or incorporate them into smoothies.

Vegetables

- Examples: Leafy greens (spinach, kale), broccoli, Brussels sprouts, and beets.

- Why They Help: Leafy greens are rich in vitamins, minerals, and antioxidants that can help combat inflammation. Broccoli contains sulforaphane, which may help reduce the symptoms of arthritis and other inflammatory conditions.

- How to Include Them: Add leafy greens to salads, smoothies, or stir-fries, and enjoy broccoli or Brussels sprouts as side dishes.

Nuts and Seeds

- Examples: Walnuts, almonds, flaxseeds, chia seeds, and hemp seeds.

- Why They Help: Nuts and seeds are reliable sources of healthy fats, fibre, and protein. Walnuts and flaxseeds are especially rich in alpha-linolenic acid (ALA), a type of omega-3 fatty acid that can help reduce inflammation.

- How to Include Them: Snack on a handful of nuts, add seeds to your yogurt or oatmeal, or include them in baked goods.

Whole Grains

- Examples: Oats, brown rice, quinoa, barley, and whole wheat.

- Why They Help: Whole grains are high in fibre, which can help reduce levels of C-reactive protein (CRP), a marker of inflammation in the blood.

- How to Include Them: Replace refined grains with whole grains in your diet. For example, choose brown rice instead of white rice or whole wheat bread instead of white bread.

Olive Oil

- Why It Helps: Extra virgin olive oil contains oleocanthal, a compound with anti-inflammatory properties like ibuprofen. It's also rich in monounsaturated fats, which are heart healthy.

- How to Include It: Use extra virgin olive oil as a base for salad dressings, drizzle it over cooked vegetables, or use it for sautéing.

Turmeric

- Why It Helps: Turmeric contains curcumin, a powerful anti-inflammatory compound that has been shown to reduce inflammation and pain in conditions like arthritis.

- How to Include It: Add turmeric to curries, soups, or smoothies. For better absorption, consume it with black pepper and a source of fat, such as olive oil.

Ginger

- Why It Helps: Ginger has anti-inflammatory and antioxidant properties that can help reduce inflammation and pain.

- How to Include It: Add fresh ginger to teas, smoothies, stir-fries, or soups.

Green Tea

- **Why It Helps:** Green tea is rich in polyphenols, particularly epigallocatechin gallate (EGCG), which has anti-inflammatory effects.

- **How to Include It:** Drink one to two cups of green tea daily to benefit from its anti-inflammatory properties.

Dark Chocolate

- **Why It Helps:** Dark chocolate contains flavonoids, which are antioxidants that have anti-inflammatory effects. Choose dark chocolate with at least 70% cocoa content for the best benefits.

- **How to Include It:** Enjoy a small piece of dark chocolate as an occasional treat.

Berries

- **Examples:** Blueberries, strawberries, raspberries, and blackberries.

- **Why They Help:** Berries are packed with antioxidants, especially anthocyanins, which have anti-inflammatory effects and can reduce inflammation.

- **How to Include Them:** Add berries to your breakfast cereal, yogurt, or smoothies, or enjoy them as a snack.

Leafy Greens

- **Examples:** Spinach, kale, Swiss chard, and collard greens.

- **Why They Help:** Leafy greens are rich in vitamins, minerals, and antioxidants that combat inflammation. They are also high in fibre, which can reduce inflammation markers in the body.

- **How to Include Them:** Use leafy greens in salads, smoothies, or as a base for dishes like stir-fries and soups.

Tomatoes

- Why They Help: Tomatoes are rich in lycopene, an antioxidant that has anti-inflammatory properties. Cooking tomatoes increases their lycopene content.

- How to Include Them: Enjoy tomatoes in salads, sauces, soups, or roasted as a side dish.

Foods to Avoid

Just as there are foods that can reduce inflammation, there are also foods that can promote inflammation and should be limited, especially if you're dealing with chronic pain. These include:

- Refined Carbohydrates: White bread, pastries, and other processed foods.

- Sugary Foods and Beverages: Soda, candy, and other sugary snacks.

- Processed Meats: Sausages, bacon, and other processed or cured meats.

- Fried Foods: Foods high in trans fats, such as fried fast food.

- Excessive Alcohol: Alcohol can increase inflammation, so it's best to limit your intake.

Incorporating anti-inflammatory foods into your diet can help reduce inflammation and may alleviate back pain. Focus on eating a variety of fruits, vegetables, whole grains, healthy fats, and lean proteins to support your overall health. Additionally, avoiding pro-inflammatory foods can further help in managing your symptoms. While diet alone may not eliminate back pain, it can be a valuable part of a comprehensive treatment plan that includes exercise, physical therapy, and other interventions as recommended by your healthcare provider.

WHICH FOODS SHOULD I AVOID BECAUSE THEY MIGHT WORSEN MY BACK PAIN?

Certain foods can promote inflammation and exacerbate back pain. If you're experiencing chronic back pain, it may be helpful to avoid or limit these foods to help reduce inflammation and manage your symptoms. Here's a list of foods to avoid or limit:

Foods and Beverages with high Sugar content
- Examples: Sodas, candies, pastries, cakes, cookies, and other sweetened snacks.

- Why to Avoid: High sugar intake can lead to increased inflammation in the body, which can exacerbate pain. Sugar can also contribute to weight gain, which can put additional strain on the back and worsen pain.

Refined Carbohydrates
- Examples: White bread, white rice, pasta, pastries, and other products made with refined flour.

- Why to Avoid: Refined carbohydrates have a high glycaemic index, causing spikes in blood sugar levels, which can lead to increased inflammation. These foods also lack fibre and essential nutrients, making them less beneficial for overall health.

Processed and Red Meats
- Examples: Bacon, sausage, hot dogs, deli meats, and red meats like beef and pork.

- Why to Avoid: Processed meats are often high in saturated fats and contain preservatives like nitrates, which can increase inflammation. Red meats, particularly those high in fat, can also contribute to inflammation and are linked to a higher risk of chronic diseases.

Fried and Fast Foods

- Examples: French fries, fried chicken, doughnuts, and other deep-fried foods.

- Why to Avoid: Fried foods are typically high in trans fats and unhealthy oils, which promote inflammation. They also contribute to weight gain, which can place additional pressure on the spine and exacerbate back pain.

Trans Fats

- Examples: Partially hydrogenated oils, margarine, some baked goods, and many processed snacks.

- Why to Avoid: Trans fats are known to increase inflammation, raise bad cholesterol levels (LDL), and lower good cholesterol levels (HDL). They are found in many processed foods and should be avoided as much as possible.

Excessive Alcohol

- Why to Avoid: Excessive alcohol consumption can increase inflammation in the body, impair healing, and contribute to nutrient deficiencies that may worsen pain. Alcohol can also contribute to weight gain, which can increase stress on the back.

High-Sodium Foods

- Examples: Canned soups, processed foods, fast foods, and salted snacks.

- Why to Avoid: High sodium intake can lead to water retention and increased blood pressure, which can contribute to inflammation. Reducing sodium can help decrease swelling and pressure on the joints and spine.

Dairy Products (for some individuals)

- Examples: Whole milk, cheese, cream, and butter.

- Why to Avoid: While dairy can be part of a healthy diet for many people, some individuals are sensitive to the proteins in dairy products, which can trigger inflammation. If you notice that dairy products worsen your pain, it may be beneficial to reduce or eliminate them.

Artificial Sweeteners and Additives

- Examples: Aspartame, saccharin, and additives found in diet sodas, sugar-free snacks, and some processed foods.

- Why to Avoid: Artificial sweeteners and additives can contribute to inflammation in some individuals. They may also cause other adverse effects, such as headaches or digestive issues, which can indirectly exacerbate pain.

To help manage and reduce back pain, it's important to avoid or limit foods that promote inflammation, such as sugary foods, refined carbohydrates, processed meats, and trans fats. Additionally, being mindful of your intake of alcohol, sodium, and certain dairy products can help minimise pain and support overall health. Replacing these foods with anti-inflammatory options like fruits, vegetables, whole grains, and healthy fats can help you better manage your back pain.

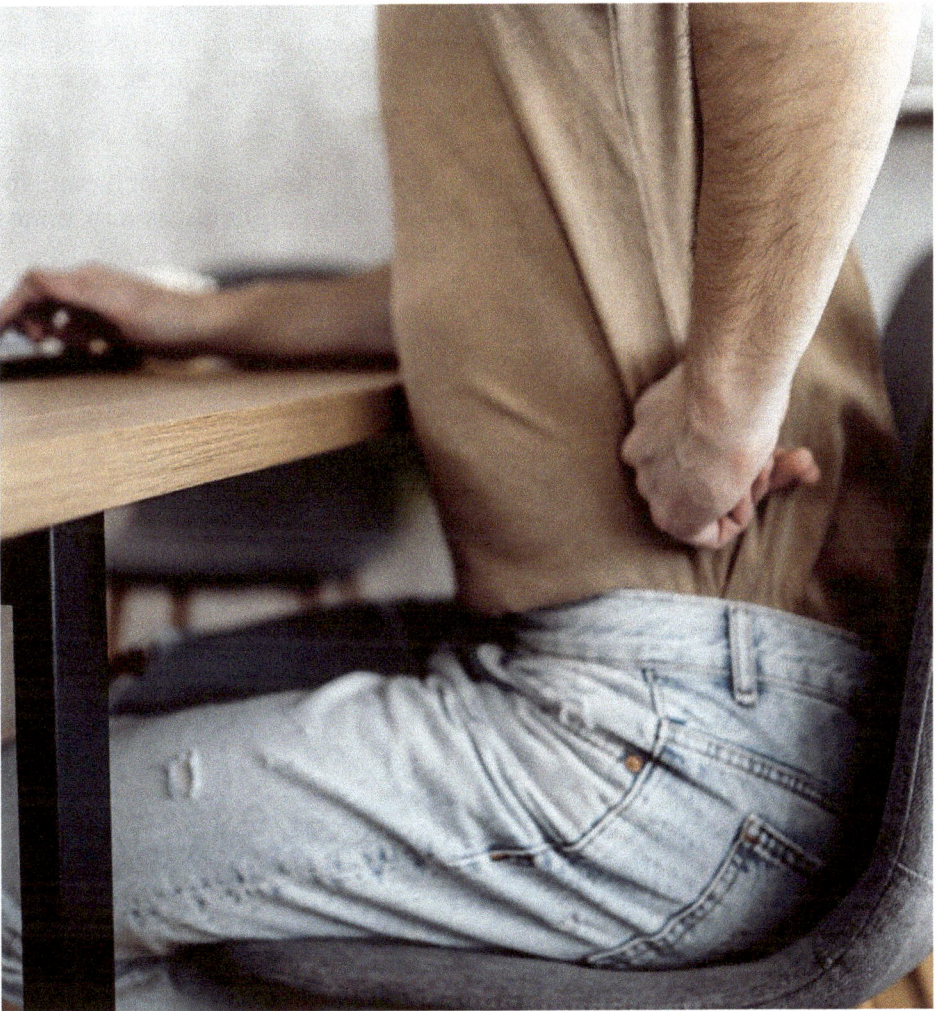

CAN MY DIET IMPACT THE HEALTH OF MY SPINE AND THE HEALING PROCESS?

Bone Health

Calcium:
- Role: Calcium is essential for maintaining strong bones, including the vertebrae in your spine. It helps in the development and maintenance of bone mass, reducing the risk of fractures and osteoporosis, which can lead to back pain.

- Sources: Dairy products (milk, yogurt, cheese), leafy green vegetables (kale, broccoli), almonds, and fortified foods (orange juice, cereals).

Vitamin D:
- Role: Vitamin D helps your body absorb calcium, making it critical for bone health. Adequate levels of vitamin D can help prevent bone-related issues such as osteoporosis.

- Sources: Sunlight exposure, fatty fish (salmon, mackerel), egg yolks, and fortified foods (milk, cereals).

Magnesium:
- Role: Magnesium is important for bone formation and plays a role in the function of muscles and nerves, which support the spine.

- Sources: Nuts and seeds (almonds, pumpkin seeds), leafy greens, whole grains, and legumes.

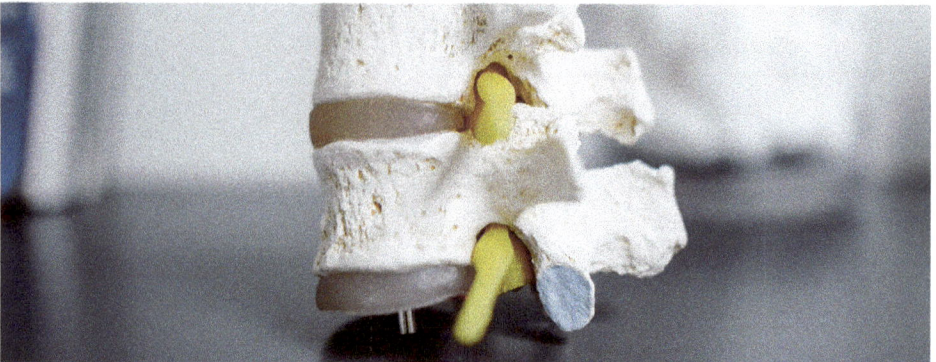

Muscle and Tissue Health

Protein:
- Role: Protein is essential for the repair and maintenance of muscles, ligaments, and other tissues that support the spine. It helps in the healing process after an injury and in maintaining muscle strength, which is crucial for spinal stability.

- Sources: Lean meats, poultry, fish, eggs, dairy products, legumes, nuts, and seeds.

Collagen:
- Role: Collagen is a protein that provides structure and strength to your bones, tendons, and ligaments. It plays a vital role in maintaining the integrity of the spinal discs.

- Sources: Bone broth, chicken, fish, egg whites, and collagen supplements

Anti-Inflammatory Nutrients

Omega-3 Fatty Acids:
- Role: Omega-3 fatty acids have anti-inflammatory properties that can help reduce inflammation and pain, which is important in the healing process of spinal injuries and conditions.

- Sources: Fatty fish (salmon, mackerel, sardines), flaxseeds, chia seeds, walnuts, and omega-3 supplements.

Antioxidants:
- Role: Antioxidants protect cells from damage caused by free radicals and reduce inflammation, which can aid in the healing process and protect spinal health.

- Sources: Fruits and vegetables, particularly berries, citrus fruits, leafy greens, and coloured vegetables like bell peppers and carrots.

Vitamin C:
- Role: Vitamin C is necessary to produce collagen, which is crucial for the repair and maintenance of connective tissues, including those in the spine.

- Sources: Citrus fruits (oranges, lemons), strawberries, bell peppers, broccoli, and kiwi.

Maintaining a Healthy Weight:
- Role: Excess body weight puts additional strain on the spine, particularly the lower back. Maintaining a healthy weight through a balanced diet can reduce pressure on the spine, improve posture, and decrease the risk of developing back pain.

- How to Achieve: Focus on a diet rich in whole foods, including fruits, vegetables, whole grains, lean proteins, and healthy fats, while limiting processed foods, sugars, and excessive caloric intake.

Hydration:
- Role: Proper hydration is essential for maintaining the elasticity and integrity of spinal discs, which cushion the vertebrae. Dehydration can lead to disc degeneration and increase the risk of injury.

- Sources: Drink plenty of water throughout the day and include hydrating foods like fruits and vegetables in your diet.

Specific Nutrients for Healing

Zinc:
- Role: Zinc is important for tissue repair and immune function, both of which are essential in the healing process after spinal injuries or surgeries.

- Sources: Meat, shellfish, legumes, seeds, and nuts.

Vitamin K:
- Role: Vitamin K is involved in bone metabolism and helps in the binding of calcium to bones, which is crucial for spinal health.

- Sources: Leafy greens (spinach, kale), broccoli, and Brussels sprouts.

Your diet plays a critical role in the health of your spine and can significantly impact the healing process after an injury or surgery. By consuming a balanced diet rich in essential nutrients like calcium, vitamin D, protein, and anti-inflammatory foods, you can support the structural integrity of your spine, reduce inflammation, and promote overall healing. Additionally, maintaining a healthy weight and staying hydrated are key factors in protecting your spine and managing back pain. Working with a healthcare provider or nutritionist can help tailor your diet to support your specific spinal health needs.

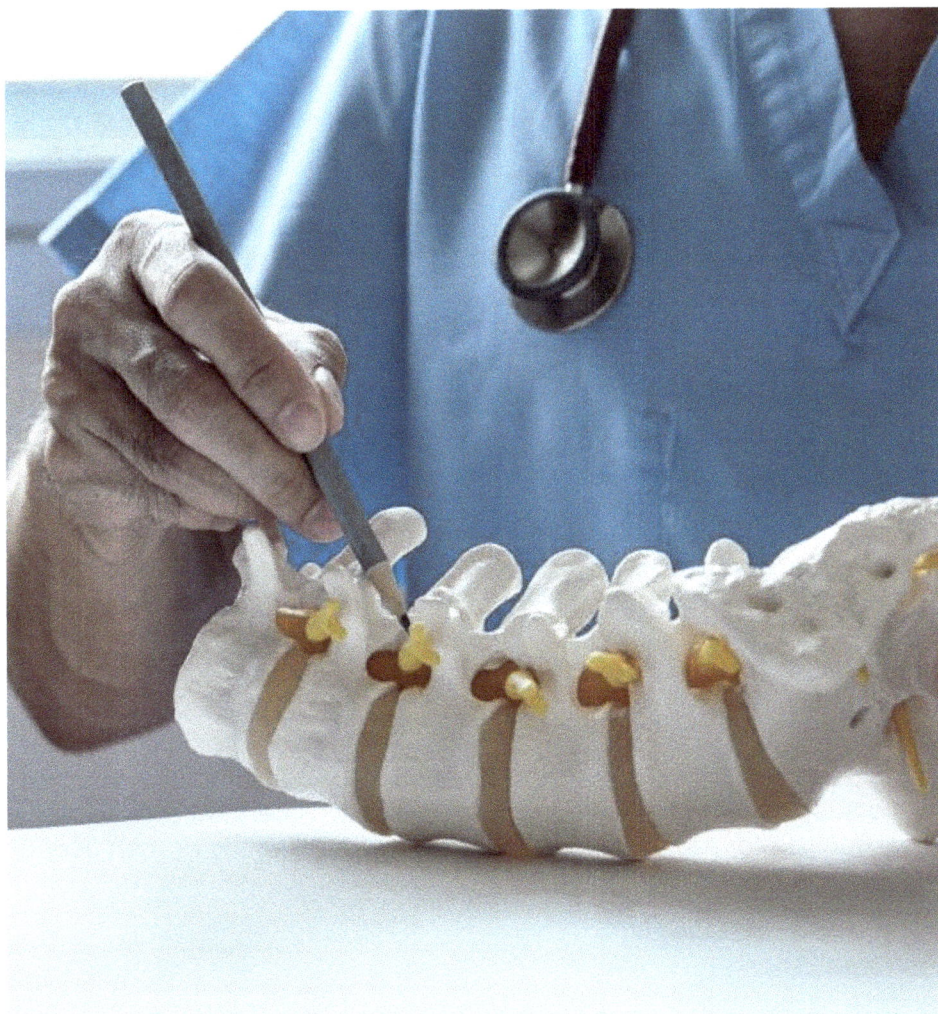

ARE THERE ANY VITAMINS OR SUPPLEMENTS THAT ARE BENEFICIAL FOR MANAGING BACK PAIN?

Certain vitamins and supplements can be beneficial for managing back pain, particularly when they address underlying issues like inflammation, bone health, or muscle function. However, it's important to consult with a healthcare provider before starting any new supplement regimen, especially if you have existing health conditions or are taking other medications. Here are some vitamins and supplements that may help with back pain:

Vitamin D
- Benefits: Vitamin D is essential for bone health, as it helps your body absorb calcium. Adequate levels of vitamin D can prevent bone-related issues such as osteoporosis, which can contribute to back pain.

- Sources: Sun exposure, fatty fish, fortified foods, and supplements.

- Supplementation: Consider taking a vitamin D supplement, especially if you have limited sun exposure or a deficiency. A typical dose is 1,000-2,000 IU daily, but higher doses may be recommended by your doctor if you are deficient.

Calcium
- Benefits: Calcium is crucial for maintaining strong bones, including the vertebrae in your spine. Adequate calcium intake can help prevent bone-related back pain and conditions like osteoporosis.

- Sources: Dairy products, leafy green vegetables, fortified foods, and supplements.

- Supplementation: If you don't get enough calcium from your diet, a supplement may be beneficial. The recommended daily intake is 1,000 mg for most adults, increasing to 1,200 mg for women over 50 and men over 70.

Magnesium
- Benefits: Magnesium plays a role in muscle function, nerve transmission, and bone health. It can help relieve muscle tension, spasms, and cramps, which are often associated with back pain.

- Sources: Nuts, seeds, leafy greens, whole grains, and supplements.

- Supplementation: Magnesium supplements are available in various forms, such as magnesium citrate or magnesium glycinate, which are more easily absorbed by the body. A typical dose ranges from 200-400 mg per day.

Omega-3 Fatty Acids
- Benefits: Omega-3 fatty acids have strong anti-inflammatory properties, which can help reduce inflammation that contributes to chronic back pain.

- Sources: Fatty fish (salmon, mackerel, sardines), flaxseeds, chia seeds, and fish oil supplements.

- Supplementation: Fish oil supplements are a common source of omega-3s. A typical dose is 1,000-3,000 mg of EPA and DHA (the active forms of omega-3s) per day.

Turmeric/Curcumin
- Benefits: Curcumin, the active compound in turmeric, has powerful anti-inflammatory and antioxidant properties. It can help reduce inflammation and pain, particularly in conditions like arthritis that affect the spine.

- Sources: Turmeric spice or curcumin supplements.

- Supplementation: Curcumin supplements are often taken in doses of 500-2,000 mg per day. Look for supplements that include black pepper extract (piperine) to enhance absorption.

Glucosamine and Chondroitin:
- Benefits: These supplements are often used to support joint health and may help alleviate pain associated with osteoarthritis, including in the spine. They are thought to help maintain cartilage and reduce inflammation.

- Sources: Supplements, typically derived from shellfish or produced synthetically.

- Supplementation: A common dose is 1,500 mg of glucosamine and 1,200 mg of chondroitin sulphate daily, taken in divided doses.

Collagen:
- Benefits: Collagen is a key component of connective tissues, including those in the spine. Supplementing with collagen may support the health of discs, tendons, and ligaments, potentially reducing pain and improving mobility.

- Sources: Bone broth, collagen-rich foods, and supplements.

- Supplementation: Collagen supplements, particularly type II collagen, are available in powder, capsule, or liquid form. A typical dose is 2.5-15 grams per day.

B Vitamins:
- Benefits: B vitamins, especially B12, B6, and folate, play a role in nerve function and can help manage nerve-related pain, such as sciatica. They may also reduce inflammation and support overall energy metabolism.

- Sources: Meat, poultry, fish, eggs, dairy, leafy greens, and supplements.

- Supplementation: B-complex vitamins are commonly taken in a single supplement containing multiple B vitamins. Dosages vary depending on the specific B vitamin, but common B-complex supplements provide around 100% of the daily value for each.

Vitamin C

- Benefits: Magnesium plays a role in muscle function, nerve transmission, and bone health. It can help relieve muscle tension, spasms, and cramps, which are often associated with back pain.

- Sources: Nuts, seeds, leafy greens, whole grains, and supplements.

- Supplementation: Magnesium supplements are available in various forms, such as magnesium citrate or magnesium glycinate, which are more easily absorbed by the body. A typical dose ranges from 200-400 mg per day.

Omega-3 Fatty Acids

- Benefits: Vitamin C is an antioxidant that supports collagen production, necessary for healthy connective tissues in the spine. It also helps reduce inflammation and supports the immune system.

- Sources: Citrus fruits, berries, bell peppers, broccoli, and supplements.

- Supplementation: A typical vitamin C supplement dose ranges from 500-1,000 mg per day.

Zinc

- Benefits: Zinc is involved in tissue repair and immune function, which are important for the healing process of spinal injuries or post-surgery recovery.

- Sources: Meat, shellfish, legumes, seeds, and nuts.

- Supplementation: A common dose of zinc supplementation is 15-30 mg per day, but higher doses should be taken under medical supervision to avoid potential side effects.

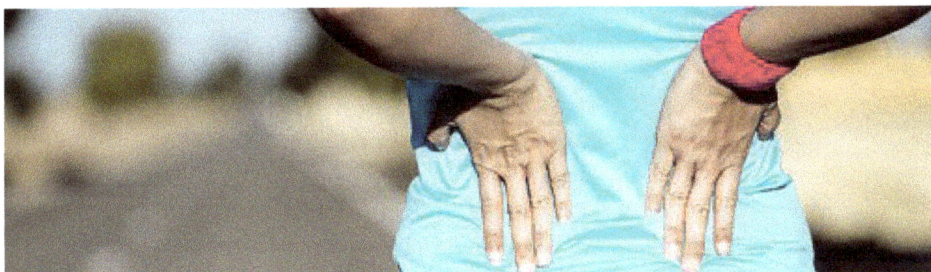

Several vitamins and supplements can support the management of back pain, particularly those that promote bone health, reduce inflammation, and support muscle function. Supplements like vitamin D, calcium, magnesium, omega-3 fatty acids, and turmeric are among the most beneficial. However, it's important to consult with a healthcare provider before starting any new supplement, as they can help determine the most appropriate supplements and dosages based on your specific needs and health status.

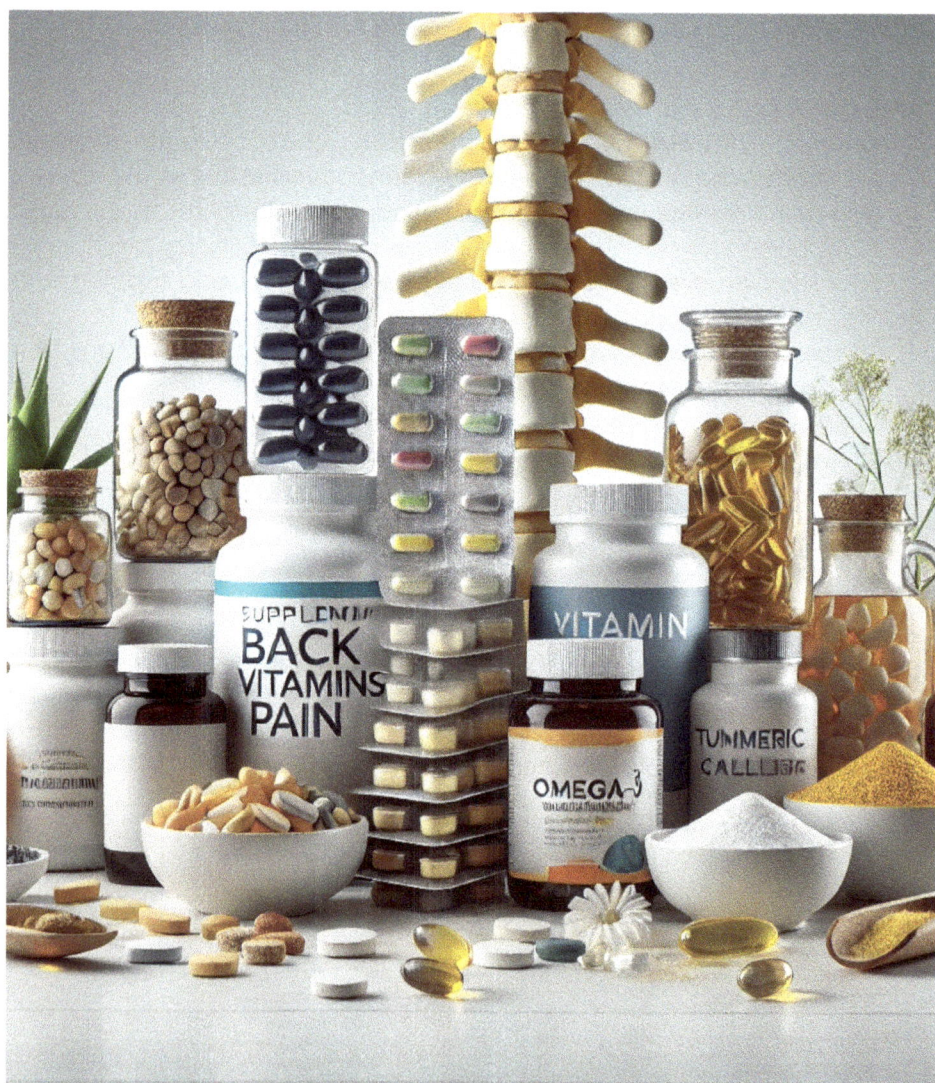

HOW DOES MAINTAINING A HEALTHY WEIGHT THROUGH DIET HELP WITH BACK PAIN MANAGEMENT?

Maintaining a healthy weight through diet plays a crucial role in managing back pain for several reasons. Excess weight, particularly around the abdomen, can put additional strain on the spine, contributing to or exacerbating back pain. Here's how a healthy weight can help manage back pain:

Reduces Pressure on the Spine

Decreased Load on Vertebrae and Discs:

- The spine supports much of the body's weight. Excess weight increases the load on the vertebrae and intervertebral discs, particularly in the lower back. This added pressure can accelerate the wear and tear of spinal structures, leading to conditions like disc degeneration or herniation, which are common causes of back pain.

- Maintaining a healthy weight reduces the overall stress on the spine, helping to prevent or alleviate pain.

Improves Posture

Balanced Weight Distribution:

- Excess weight, especially in the abdominal area, can shift your center of gravity forward, causing your pelvis to tilt and your lower back to curve more than usual (a condition known as lordosis). This imbalance can lead to poor posture, which strains the muscles, ligaments, and joints in the back.

- A healthy weight helps maintain proper posture by ensuring that your body's weight is evenly distributed, reducing strain on the back muscles and spine.

Reduces Inflammation

Lower Levels of Inflammatory Markers:
- Excess body fat, particularly visceral fat (fat around the organs), is associated with increased levels of inflammatory markers like C-reactive protein (CRP). Chronic inflammation can exacerbate back pain, especially in conditions like arthritis or disc disease.

- A diet that promotes weight loss can help reduce body fat and lower inflammation, which may, in turn, alleviate pain.

Decreases the Risk of Related Health Conditions

Prevents Weight-Related Conditions:
- Obesity is a risk factor for several conditions that can cause or worsen back pain, including osteoarthritis, degenerative disc disease, and spinal stenosis. It's also associated with a higher risk of developing diabetes and cardiovascular disease, which can indirectly contribute to back pain through poor circulation and nerve health.

- Maintaining a healthy weight reduces the risk of these conditions, thereby decreasing the likelihood of developing back pain or worsening existing pain.

Enhances Mobility and Flexibility

Easier Movement:
- Excess weight can limit mobility and make physical activity more difficult, leading to a sedentary lifestyle. Lack of movement can weaken muscles, reduce flexibility, and increase stiffness, all of which can contribute to back pain.

- A healthy weight makes it easier to stay active, which is essential for maintaining strong and flexible muscles that support the spine.

Supports Effective Pain Management Strategies

Improves Response to Treatment:
- Weight loss can enhance the effectiveness of other back pain management strategies, such as physical therapy, exercise, and medication. For instance, losing weight can make physical activity less painful, allowing you to engage more fully in rehabilitation exercises that strengthen the back and core muscles.

- Additionally, weight loss may reduce the need for medications or lower the required dose, minimising the risk of side effects.

Promotes Overall Health

Better Nutrient Intake:
- A diet focused on maintaining a healthy weight is typically rich in fruits, vegetables, whole grains, lean proteins, and healthy fats. These foods provide essential nutrients that support bone and muscle health, reduce inflammation, and promote overall well-being, all of which are important for managing back pain.

- Proper nutrition also supports the immune system and the body's natural healing processes, which can help with recovery from back injuries or surgeries.

So, maintaining a healthy weight through diet is a key component of back pain management. It reduces pressure on the spine, improves posture, decreases inflammation, and lowers the risk of related health conditions. Additionally, a healthy weight supports better mobility and enhances the effectiveness of other pain management strategies. By focusing on a balanced diet that promotes weight loss or weight maintenance, you can significantly reduce your risk of back pain and improve your overall quality of life.

IS THERE A CONNECTION BETWEEN DEHYDRATION AND INCREASED BACK PAIN, AND HOW MUCH WATER SHOULD I DRINK DAILY?

There is a connection between dehydration and increased back pain. Dehydration can impact the health of your spinal discs and muscles, which are critical components of a healthy back. Here's how dehydration can contribute to back pain:

Spinal Disc Health

Role of Intervertebral Discs:
- The intervertebral discs act as cushions between the vertebrae in your spine, allowing for flexibility and absorbing shock. These discs are composed of water, which helps them maintain their shape, flexibility, and cushioning ability.

Impact of Dehydration:
- When you are dehydrated, the intervertebral discs can lose some of their water content, which can cause them to shrink and reduce their ability to cushion the spine. This dehydration can lead to increased pressure on the spine, reduced disc height, and an increased risk of disc degeneration or herniation, all of which can cause or exacerbate back pain.

Muscle Function

Muscle Cramps and Spasms:
- The intervertebral discs act as cushions between the vertebrae in your spine, allowing for flexibility and absorbing shock. These discs are composed of water, which helps them maintain their shape, flexibility, and cushioning ability.

Reduced Flexibility:
- Dehydration can also reduce the flexibility of muscles, ligaments, and tendons, making the back more susceptible to strains and injuries.

Joint Lubrication

Synovial Fluid:
- Proper hydration is important for the body to produce synovial fluid, which lubricates the joints, including those in the spine. Dehydration can reduce the amount of this fluid, leading to increased friction in the joints and contributing to joint pain and stiffness.

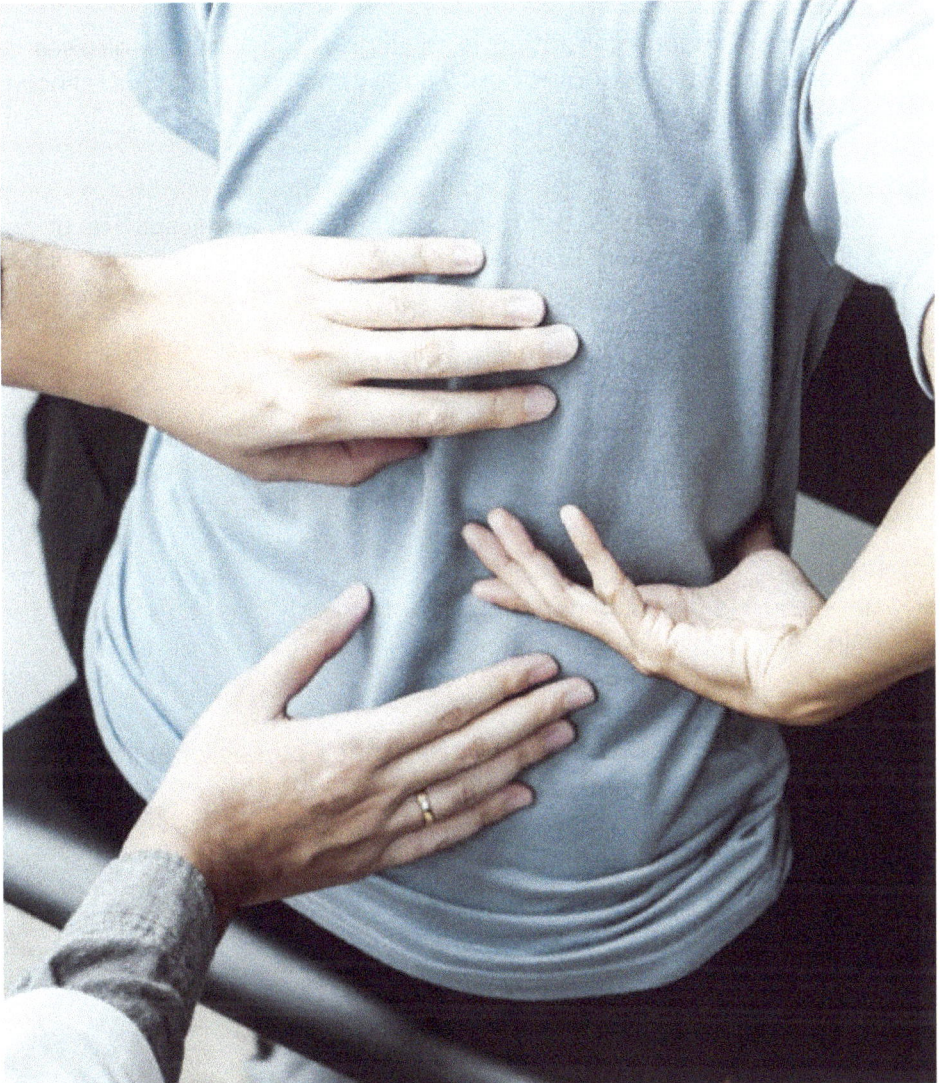

HOW MUCH WATER SHOULD YOU DRINK DAILY?

The amount of water you should drink daily can vary based on factors like your body size, activity level, climate, and overall health. However, general guidelines can help ensure you stay adequately hydrated:

General Guidelines

8x8 Rule:
- A common recommendation is to drink eight 8-ounce glasses of water a day, which equals about 2 litres or half a gallon. This is known as the "8x8 rule."

Individual Needs:
- Some health experts recommend drinking more water, such as about 3 litres (approximately 13 cups) for men and 2.2 litres (about 9 cups) for women, based on the Institute of Medicine's guidelines.

Factors That May Increase Your Water Needs

Physical Activity:
- If you are physically active or sweat heavily, you will need to drink more water to replace the fluids lost during exercise.

Climate:
- Hot or humid climates can increase your body's need for water due to increased sweating.

Climate:
- Certain health conditions, such as kidney stones or urinary tract infections, may require you to drink more water.

Pregnancy and Breastfeeding:
- Pregnant and breastfeeding women typically need more fluids to stay hydrated.

Listening to Your Body

Thirst and Urine Colour:
* Pay attention to your body's signals, such as thirst, and monitor the colour of your urine. Light yellow or pale straw-coloured urine indicates good hydration, while dark yellow or amber-coloured urine can be a sign of dehydration.

In other words, lack of water and subsequent dehydration can contribute to increased back pain by affecting the health of your spinal discs, muscles, and joints. Ensuring that you drink enough water daily is important for maintaining spinal health, reducing the risk of back pain, and supporting overall well-being. While general guidelines suggest drinking about 2-3 litres of water a day, individual needs may vary, so it's important to listen to your body and adjust your intake accordingly. If you have specific health concerns or conditions, it's advisable to consult with a healthcare provider to determine the best hydration strategy for you.

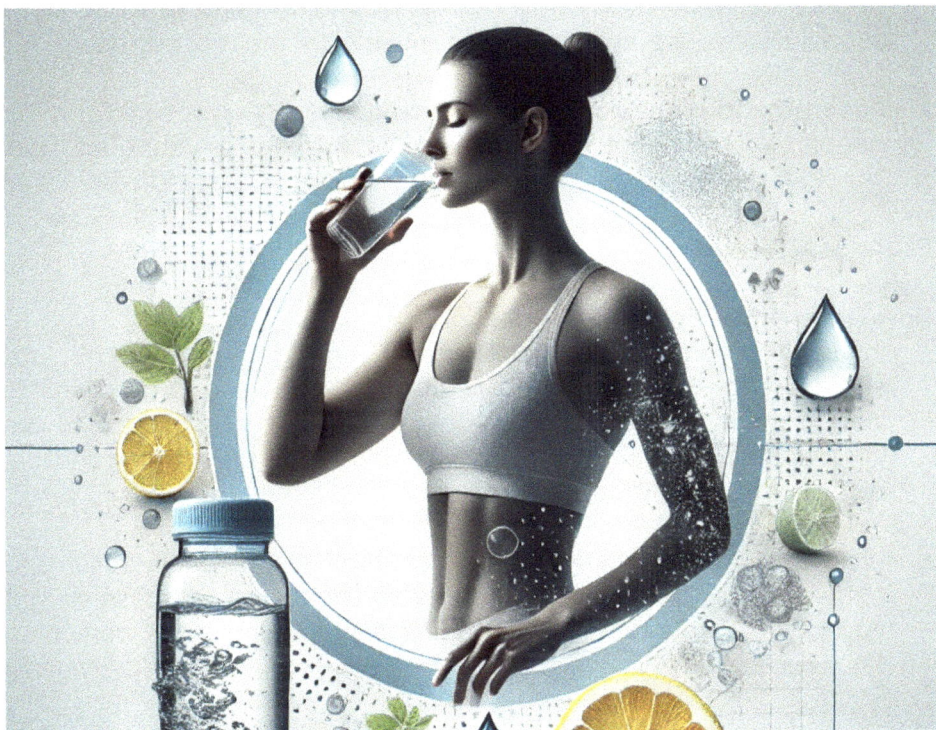

CAN CERTAIN FOODS OR BEVERAGES TRIGGER BACK PAIN FLARE-UPS, SUCH AS CAFFEINE OR PROCESSED FOODS?

Certain foods and beverages can potentially trigger back pain flare-ups, particularly if they contribute to inflammation, dehydration, or weight gain. Here's a closer look at some of the common dietary triggers that might exacerbate back pain:

Caffeine

How It Might Trigger Back Pain:

*   Dehydration: Caffeine is a diuretic, meaning it can increase urine production and potentially lead to dehydration if consumed in excess. Dehydration can reduce the water content in your spinal discs and muscles, which may increase the likelihood of pain or discomfort.

*   Muscle Tension: Caffeine can also increase muscle tension and anxiety in some individuals, which might exacerbate back pain, especially if your pain is related to muscle tightness or spasms.

*   **Recommendation:** Moderate caffeine consumption is safe for most people. If you suspect that caffeine is contributing to your back pain, consider reducing your intake and monitoring your symptoms.

Processed Foods

How They Might Trigger Back Pain:

*   Inflammation: Processed foods are often high in unhealthy fats, sugars, and refined carbohydrates, all of which can promote inflammation in the body. Chronic inflammation can exacerbate conditions like arthritis, disc degeneration, and other inflammatory disorders that contribute to back pain.

*   Weight Gain: Processed foods are typically calorie-dense and nutrient-poor, which can contribute to weight gain. Excess weight can place additional strain on the spine, leading to or worsening back pain.

Examples of Processed Foods to Limit:

- Fast foods, packaged snacks (chips, cookies), sugary cereals, processed meats (hot dogs, sausages), and frozen meals.

- **Recommendation:** Focus on a diet rich in whole, unprocessed foods such as fruits, vegetables, lean proteins, whole grains, and healthy fats to reduce inflammation and support overall health.

High Sugar content Foods and Beverages

How They Might Trigger Back Pain:

- Inflammation: High sugar intake can lead to increased levels of inflammatory markers in the body, which can exacerbate pain, particularly in people with inflammatory conditions like arthritis.

- Insulin Resistance: Excessive sugar consumption can contribute to insulin resistance and metabolic syndrome, both of which are associated with increased inflammation and a higher risk of chronic pain conditions.

Examples to Limit:

- Sodas, candy, baked goods, sugary cereals, and desserts.

- **Recommendation:** Reduce your intake of added sugars and opt for natural sources of sweetness like fruits when possible.

High-Sodium Foods

How They Might Trigger Back Pain:

- Fluid Retention: High sodium intake can cause your body to retain water, leading to bloating and increased pressure on the spine and joints. This can exacerbate pain, particularly in the lower back.

- Increased Blood Pressure: Excess sodium can also contribute to high blood pressure, which is associated with a higher risk of pain and inflammation.

Examples to Limit:
- Canned soups, processed snacks, fast food, salted nuts, and cured meats.

- **Recommendation:** Choose low-sodium or no-added-salt options and use herbs and spices to flavour your food instead of salt.

Alcohol

How It Might Trigger Back Pain:
- Dehydration: Alcohol is a diuretic, which can lead to dehydration. As with caffeine, dehydration can contribute to back pain by reducing the hydration of spinal discs and muscles.

- Inflammation: Alcohol can promote inflammation and may worsen pain, particularly if consumed in excess.

- Interference with Sleep: Alcohol can disrupt sleep patterns, and poor sleep is often linked to increased perception of pain.

- **Recommendation:** Limit alcohol consumption and ensure you stay hydrated by drinking plenty of water.

Dairy Products (for Some Individuals)

How They Might Trigger Back Pain:
- Inflammatory Response: While dairy products can be part of a healthy diet, some individuals are sensitive to the proteins in dairy (such as casein), which can trigger an inflammatory response. This inflammation may exacerbate back pain, particularly in people with lactose intolerance or dairy allergies.

- **Recommendation:** If you suspect dairy may be contributing to your back pain, consider reducing or eliminating it from your diet and monitoring how your body responds. Choose non-dairy alternatives like almond milk, soy milk, or oat milk.

Artificial Sweeteners and Additives

How They Might Trigger Back Pain:
- Inflammatory Response: Some artificial sweeteners and food additives can trigger an inflammatory response or other adverse effects in sensitive individuals. For example, aspartame has been reported to cause headaches, joint pain, and other symptoms in some people.

Examples to Limit:
- Diet sodas, sugar-free candies, and low-calorie processed foods that contain artificial sweeteners like aspartame, saccharin, and sucralose.

- **Recommendation:** Consider using natural sweeteners like honey, maple syrup, or stevia in moderation, and reduce consumption of artificially sweetened products.

Certain foods and beverages, such as those high in sugar, sodium, unhealthy fats, and artificial additives, can potentially trigger back pain flare-ups by promoting inflammation, dehydration, or muscle tension. By focusing on a balanced diet rich in whole, unprocessed foods and staying hydrated, you can help manage your back pain more effectively. If you notice specific foods or drinks seem to worsen your symptoms, consider limiting or avoiding them and consult with a healthcare provider or nutritionist for personalised dietary advice.

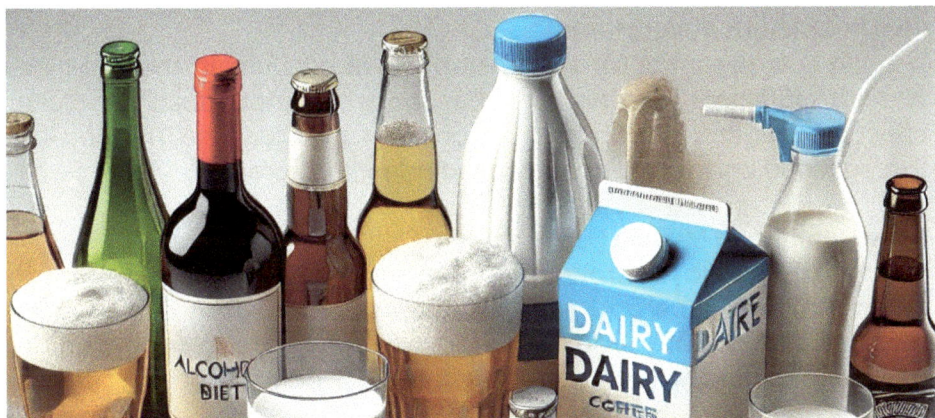

HOW IMPORTANT IS CALCIUM AND VITAMIN D IN PREVENTING BONE-RELATED BACK ISSUES, AND WHAT ARE THE BEST DIETARY SOURCES?

Calcium and vitamin D are essential nutrients that play a critical role in maintaining bone health and preventing bone-related back issues, such as osteoporosis, fractures, and degenerative spine conditions. Here's why they are important:

Calcium

Role in Bone Health:
- Calcium is the primary mineral found in bones and is essential for maintaining their strength and density. It helps in the development and maintenance of bone mass throughout life. Adequate calcium intake is crucial for preventing osteoporosis, a condition where bones become weak and brittle, increasing the risk of fractures, including those in the spine.

Impact on Spinal Health:
- The vertebrae in your spine are susceptible to fractures if your bones are weakened due to calcium deficiency. Ensuring adequate calcium intake helps maintain the structural integrity of your spine and reduces the risk of bone-related back pain.

Vitamin D

Role in Calcium Absorption:
Vitamin D is essential for the absorption of calcium in the intestines. Without sufficient vitamin D, your body cannot absorb calcium effectively, regardless of how much calcium you consume. This can lead to weakened bones and an increased risk of fractures.

Bone Health and Muscle Function:
Vitamin D also plays a role in muscle function, which is important for maintaining balance and reducing the risk of falls that could lead to fractures. Inadequate vitamin D levels can contribute to bone pain and muscle weakness, which can exacerbate back pain.

BEST DIETARY SOURCES OF CALCIUM AND VITAMIN D

Calcium-Rich Foods

Dairy Products

Examples: Milk, yogurt, cheese.

Why They Help: Dairy products are among the best sources of calcium. They are also often fortified with vitamin D, making them doubly beneficial for bone health.

Leafy Green Vegetables

Examples: Kale, broccoli, collard greens, bok choy.

Why They Help: Leafy greens are good plant-based sources of calcium, though they contain lower amounts than dairy products. They are particularly important for those following a vegan or lactose-intolerant diet.

Fortified Foods

Examples: Fortified plant-based milks (almond, soy, rice), fortified orange juice, fortified cereals.

Why They Help: Many plant-based milk alternatives and other products are fortified with calcium to help meet daily intake needs.

Fish with Edible Bones

Examples: Canned salmon, sardines.

Why They Help: These fish are excellent sources of calcium because their edible bones are rich in the mineral.

Other Sources

Examples: Almonds, tofu, tahini (sesame paste).

Why They Help: These foods offer additional plant-based calcium sources, particularly beneficial for those who avoid dairy.

Vitamin D-Rich Foods

Fatty Fish

Examples: Salmon, mackerel, sardines, tuna.

Why They Help: Fatty fish are among the best natural sources of vitamin D. They also provide omega-3 fatty acids, which have anti-inflammatory properties.

Fortified Foods

Examples: Fortified milk (dairy and non-dairy), fortified orange juice, fortified cereals.

Why They Help: Many foods are fortified with vitamin D, providing an accessible way to increase your intake, especially in regions with limited sunlight.

Egg Yolks

Why They Help: Egg yolks contain small amounts of vitamin D, contributing to your overall intake.

Mushrooms

Why They Help: Some mushrooms, especially those exposed to sunlight or UV light, can be a good plant-based source of vitamin D.

Sunlight Exposure

Importance of Sunlight

The body can produce vitamin D naturally when the skin is exposed to sunlight. Spending time outdoors in the sun (without sunscreen for short periods) can help maintain adequate vitamin D levels, particularly in the summer months.

Considerations

In regions with limited sunlight, especially during the winter months, or for individuals with limited outdoor activity, supplementation or fortified foods may be necessary to maintain adequate vitamin D levels.

Both Calcium and vitamin D are crucial for preventing bone-related health conditions and more important back issues by ensuring strong and healthy bones and proper muscle function. A diet rich in these nutrients, combined with adequate sunlight exposure, can significantly reduce the risk of conditions like osteoporosis and fractures, which are common causes of back pain. If you are concerned about your calcium or vitamin D intake, or if you have specific health conditions, it's a good idea to consult with a healthcare provider who can recommend the appropriate dietary changes or supplements based on your individual needs.

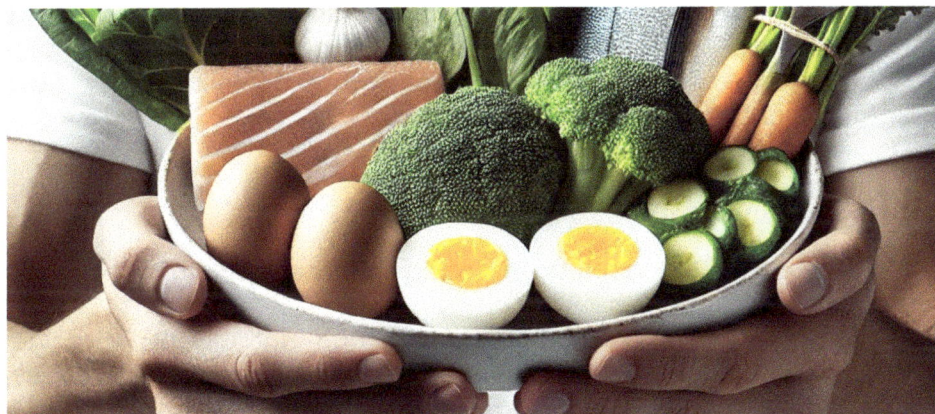

ARE THERE ANY DIETARY CHANGES I CAN MAKE TO IMPROVE MY OVERALL JOINT HEALTH AND POTENTIALLY REDUCE BACK PAIN?

Making specific dietary changes can significantly improve overall joint health and potentially reduce back pain. A diet that focuses on anti-inflammatory foods, adequate nutrients for bone and joint support, and maintaining a healthy weight can contribute to better joint function and alleviate pain. Here are some dietary strategies you can implement:

Increase Anti-Inflammatory Foods

Fatty Fish

Examples: Salmon, mackerel, sardines, and trout.

Benefits: Rich in omega-3 fatty acids, which have potent anti-inflammatory effects that can help reduce joint pain and stiffness, especially in conditions like arthritis.

Fruits and Vegetables

Examples: Berries (blueberries, strawberries), leafy greens (spinach, kale), and colourful vegetables (bell peppers, carrots).

Benefits: High in antioxidants, vitamins, and minerals that help combat inflammation and support overall joint health. Berries in particular, are rich in anthocyanins, which have anti-inflammatory properties.

Nuts and Seeds:

Examples: Walnuts, flaxseeds, chia seeds, and almonds.

Benefits: Provide healthy fats and antioxidants that can reduce inflammation and support joint health. Walnuts and flaxseeds are also good sources of omega-3 fatty acids.

Olive Oil

Benefits: Extra virgin olive oil contains oleocanthal, a compound with anti-inflammatory effects similar to ibuprofen. It also provides heart-healthy monounsaturated fats.

Usage: Use olive oil as a base for salad dressings, drizzle over cooked vegetables, or use for sautéing.

Incorporate Bone-Building Nutrients

Calcium

The body can produce vitamin D naturally when the skin is exposed to sunlight. Spending time outdoors in the sun (without sunscreen for short periods) can help maintain adequate vitamin D levels, particularly in the summer months.

Vitamin D

Examples: Fatty fish, fortified foods (milk, orange juice), egg yolks, and mushrooms exposed to sunlight.

Benefits: Facilitates calcium absorption and bone health and may reduce the risk of osteoporosis. Adequate vitamin D levels are crucial for maintaining bone density and overall skeletal health.

Magnesium

Examples: Nuts (almonds, cashews), seeds (pumpkin seeds), whole grains, and leafy greens.

Benefits: Supports bone health and helps regulate muscle and nerve function, which is important for maintaining proper joint function and reducing muscle spasms that can contribute to back pain.

Support Cartilage and Joint Tissue

Collagen

Examples: Bone broth, collagen-rich foods, and collagen supplements.

Benefits: Collagen is a key component of cartilage, tendons, and ligaments. Supplementing with collagen can support joint health and reduce pain associated with degenerative joint conditions.

Glucosamine and Chondroitin

Sources: Typically found in supplements, but also in shellfish (glucosamine) and animal cartilage.

Benefits: These compounds are involved in the maintenance and repair of cartilage. They may help reduce joint pain and improve mobility, especially in people with osteoarthritis.

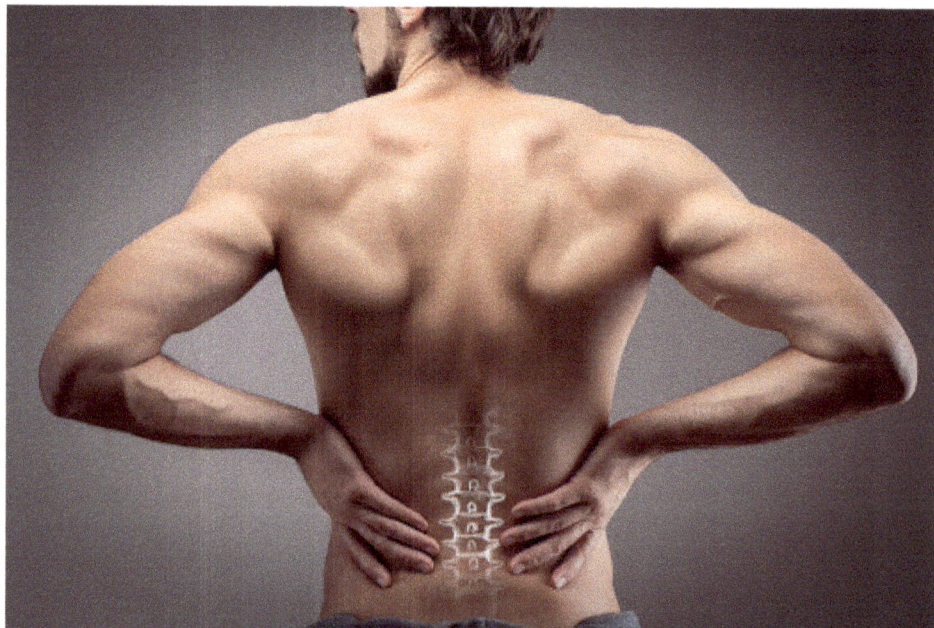

Maintain a Healthy Weight

Role in Joint Health:
- Excess weight puts additional strain on the joints, particularly the knees, hips, and lower back. Maintaining a healthy weight through a balanced diet can reduce pressure on these joints, decrease inflammation, and lower the risk of developing or worsening back pain.

Strategies:
- Focus on portion control, choose nutrient-dense foods, and avoid excessive consumption of high-calorie, low-nutrient foods. Include plenty of fruits, vegetables, lean proteins, and whole grains in your diet to support weight management.

Stay Hydrated

Importance for Joint Health:
- Proper hydration is essential for maintaining the lubrication of joints and the health of spinal discs. Dehydration can lead to decreased synovial fluid, which cushions joints, and can cause the discs in the spine to lose their elasticity and cushioning ability, increasing the risk of back pain.

Recommendations:
- Aim to drink at least 8 glasses of water a day, and more if you are physically active or live in a hot climate. Include water-rich foods like fruits and vegetables in your diet.

Limit Foods That Promote Inflammation

Sugary Foods and Beverages:
- Examples: Sodas, candies, pastries.

- Impact: High sugar intake can increase inflammation and contribute to joint pain.

Processed Foods:
- Examples: Fast foods, packaged snacks, processed meats.

- Impact: These foods are often high in unhealthy fats, sodium, and additives that can promote inflammation and negatively affect joint health.

Refined Carbohydrates:
- Examples: White bread, white rice, and pastries.

- Impact: Refined carbs can cause spikes in blood sugar levels and increase inflammation, which may exacerbate joint pain.

Consider Anti-Inflammatory Supplements

Omega-3 Fatty Acids:
- Benefits: Help reduce inflammation and support joint health.

- Sources: Fish oil supplements or algae-based omega-3 supplements (for vegetarians/vegans).

Turmeric/Curcumin:
- Benefits: Curcumin, the active compound in turmeric, has strong anti-inflammatory and antioxidant properties that can help reduce joint pain.

- Usage: Consider taking a curcumin supplement, especially one combined with black pepper (peperine) to enhance absorption.

Dietary changes can play a significant role in improving joint health and potentially reducing back pain. By focusing on anti-inflammatory foods, ensuring adequate intake of bone-building nutrients, maintaining a healthy weight, and staying hydrated, you can support your joints and reduce the risk of pain. Additionally, limiting foods that promote inflammation can further enhance these benefits. If you're considering supplements or making significant dietary changes, it's always a good idea to consult with a healthcare provider or a nutritionist to tailor your diet to your specific needs and conditions.

HOW STRESS IS INFLUENCING BACK PAIN

These questions highlight the relationship between stress and back pain, especially during the acute phase, and explore practical ways to manage stress to improve pain outcomes.

HOW DOES STRESS AFFECT MY BACK PAIN, AND WHY IS IT IMPORTANT TO MANAGE IT DURING THE ACUTE PHASE?

Stress can significantly impact back pain, and managing it during the acute phase is crucial for several reasons:

How Stress Affects Back Pain

- Muscle Tension: Stress triggers the body's "fight or flight" response, leading to muscle tension. This tension can increase tightness in the back muscles, exacerbating pain or leading to muscle spasms.

- Inflammation: Stress hormones, like cortisol, can contribute to increased inflammation in the body. Inflammation is often associated with pain, particularly in the case of acute back pain, where tissue damage or irritation is present.

- Pain Perception: Stress can alter how pain is perceived. High stress levels can heighten your sensitivity to pain, making back pain feel more intense than it might otherwise be.

- Behavioural Factors: Stress can affect sleep quality, posture, and physical activity levels. Poor sleep can impair healing, while stress-induced poor posture and reduced activity can strain the back further.

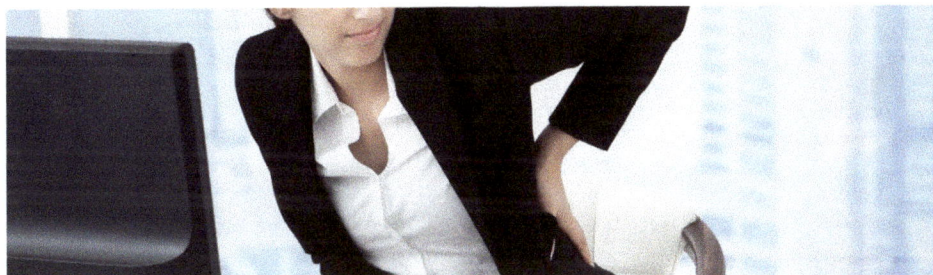

Importance of Managing Stress During the Acute Phase

- Facilitates Healing: Reducing stress helps in lowering muscle tension and inflammation, which can accelerate recovery from acute back pain.

- Prevents Chronicity: If stress is not managed, acute back pain can become chronic. The longer pain persists, the more likely it is that the body will develop a pain memory, making future episodes more severe and harder to treat.

- Improves Coping Mechanisms: Managing stress early can improve your ability to cope with pain, leading to better outcomes. It helps in maintaining a positive outlook and prevents the development of anxiety or depression, which are often linked with chronic pain conditions.

- Enhances Overall Treatment: Managing stress can make other treatments (like physical therapy, medication, or exercise) more effective. When the body is less tense and inflamed, it responds better to these interventions.

Addressing stress early during back pain can be a critical component of both short-term recovery and long-term health.

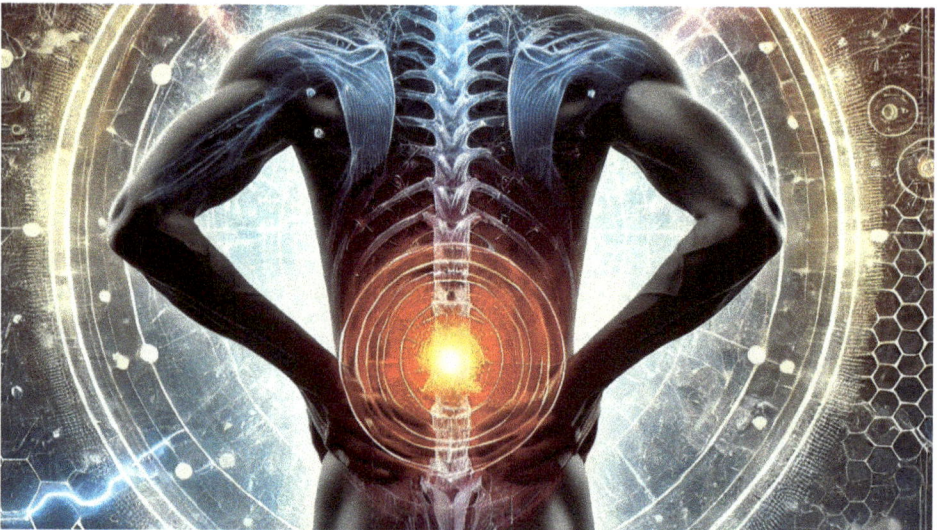

WHAT ARE THE MOST EFFECTIVE STRESS-RELIEF TECHNIQUES I CAN USE TO HELP REDUCE MY BACK PAIN?

Reducing stress can play a key role in managing and alleviating back pain. Here are some of the most effective stress-relief techniques that you can use:

Mindfulness Meditation:
- How It Helps: Mindfulness meditation involves focusing on the present moment and can help reduce the perception of pain and stress. It promotes relaxation and decreases the body's stress response.

- How to Do It: Sit or lie down in a comfortable position. Focus on your breath or a particular sensation in your body. If your mind wanders, gently bring it back to your breath. Start with just a few minutes a day and gradually increase the time.

Deep Breathing Exercises:
- How It Helps: Deep breathing stimulates the parasympathetic nervous system, promoting relaxation and reducing muscle tension in the back.

- How to Do It: Try diaphragmatic breathing—breathe in deeply through your nose, allowing your abdomen to expand rather than your chest. Exhale slowly through your mouth. Practice for 5-10 minutes a few times a day.

Progressive Muscle Relaxation (PMR):
- How It Helps: PMR involves tensing and then slowly releasing different muscle groups in the body. This can help reduce overall muscle tension and pain.

- How to Do It: Start with your feet and work your way up to your head, tensing each muscle group for 5 seconds and then relaxing it for 30 seconds.

Yoga and Stretching

- How It Helps: Yoga combines physical postures, breathing exercises, and meditation, helping reduce stress and improve flexibility and muscle strength, which can relieve back pain.

- How to Do It: Gentle yoga poses like Child's Pose, Cat-Cow Stretch, and Downward Dog can be particularly beneficial. Consider following a yoga video or attending a class designed for back pain relief.

Exercise and Physical Activity

- How It Helps: Regular physical activity reduces stress by releasing endorphins, which are natural painkillers and mood elevators. It also helps keep the back muscles strong and flexible.

- How to Do It: Engage in low-impact exercises like walking, swimming, or cycling for 30 minutes most days of the week. Ensure that the exercise intensity is appropriate for your fitness level and current back condition.

Cognitive Behavioural Therapy (CBT)

- How It Helps: CBT helps you identify and change negative thought patterns that can increase stress and pain. It teaches coping strategies to manage pain more effectively.

- How to Do It: You can work with a therapist who specialises in CBT, or there are self-help resources and apps available that can guide you through CBT techniques.

Visualisation and Guided Imagery

- How It Helps: Visualisation techniques involve imagining a peaceful scene or outcome, which can reduce stress and the perception of pain.

- How to Do It: Close your eyes and picture a calming place, like a beach or forest. Focus on the sensory details, like the sound of waves or the smell of pine trees. Spend 5-10 minutes in this mental space.

Biofeedback:
- How It Helps: Biofeedback teaches you to control physiological functions such as muscle tension and heart rate. It can be particularly effective for reducing stress-related muscle tension in the back.

- How to Do It: Biofeedback typically requires a professional or a specialised device. Sensors monitor physiological functions, and you learn to control these through relaxation techniques.

Adequate Sleep:
- How It Helps: Poor sleep can increase stress and make pain worse. Good sleep hygiene practices can reduce stress and improve recovery.

- How to Do It: Establish a regular sleep schedule, create a relaxing bedtime routine, and ensure your sleeping environment is comfortable and conducive to sleep.

Social Support and Communication:
- How It Helps: Talking with friends, family, or a therapist can reduce stress by providing emotional support and perspective.

- How to Do It: Regularly connect with supportive people in your life. Consider joining a support group for people dealing with chronic pain.

Incorporating a combination of these techniques into your daily routine can significantly reduce stress and help alleviate back pain.

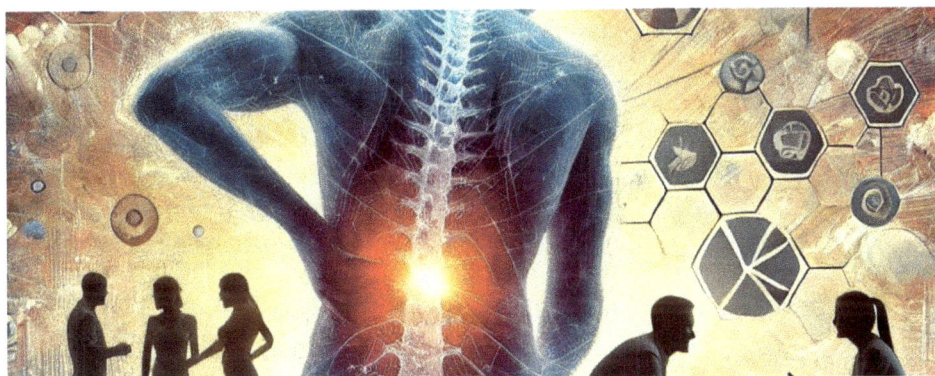

CAN DEEP BREATHING EXERCISES OR MEDITATION HELP RELIEVE MY BACK PAIN, AND HOW SHOULD I PRACTICE THEM?

Deep breathing exercises and meditation can be effective in relieving back pain, especially when stress is a contributing factor. Both techniques promote relaxation, reduce muscle tension, and enhance your overall pain management ability.

How Deep Breathing Exercises Help Relieve Back Pain:

- Reduces Muscle Tension: Deep breathing helps relax the muscles, including those in your back. When you're stressed, your muscles tend to tense up, which can exacerbate back pain.

- Lowers Stress Levels: Deep breathing activates the parasympathetic nervous system, which counteracts the body's stress response, leading to lower cortisol levels and reduced inflammation.

- Improves Oxygenation: Better oxygen flow to muscles and tissues promotes healing and reduces discomfort.

How to Practice Deep Breathing for Back Pain Relief:

Diaphragmatic Breathing:
- Find a Comfortable Position: Sit or lie down in a comfortable position, ensuring your back is well-supported.

- Inhale Slowly: Place one hand on your chest and the other on your abdomen. Breathe in slowly through your nose, allowing your abdomen (not your chest) to rise as you fill your lungs with air.

- Exhale Slowly: Exhale slowly through your mouth, allowing your abdomen to fall as you expel the air. Aim for a slow, steady rhythm.

- Practice Regularly: Try this for 5-10 minutes, 2-3 times a day, or whenever you feel stressed or notice your back pain intensifying.

4-7-8 Breathing Technique:
- Inhale for 4 Seconds: Breathe in quietly through your nose for a count of four.

- Hold for 7 Seconds: Hold your breath for a count of seven.

- Exhale for 8 Seconds: Exhale completely through your mouth, making a whooshing sound, for a count of eight.

- Repeat: Repeat this cycle 3-4 times, focusing on the breath and the count. This technique is particularly useful for calming the nervous system.

How Meditation Helps Relieve Back Pain:
- Alters Pain Perception: Meditation, particularly mindfulness meditation helps you become more aware of your body and thoughts, which can change how you perceive pain therefore reducing its intensity.

- Reduces Stress: Meditation lowers stress levels by promoting relaxation and reducing the production of stress hormones like cortisol.

- Improves Coping Skills: Regular meditation practice can improve your overall ability to cope with pain and discomfort, making it easier to manage chronic conditions like back pain.

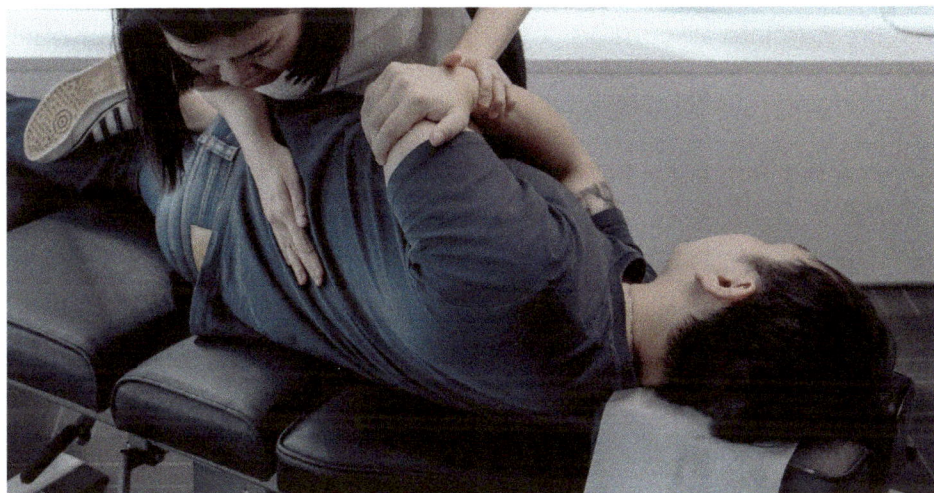

How to Practice Meditation for Back Pain Relief:

Mindfulness Meditation:
- Find a Quiet Space: Sit or lie down in a quiet, comfortable space.

- Focus on Your Breath: Close your eyes and begin to focus on your breathing. Notice the sensation of the breath entering and leaving your body.

- Acknowledge Discomfort: If you notice pain or discomfort in your back, acknowledge it without judgment, and try to observe it as a neutral sensation.

- Stay Present: Whenever your mind wanders, gently bring your focus back to your breath or body sensations.

- Duration: Start with just 5-10 minutes a day, gradually increasing the time as you become more comfortable with the practice.

Body Scan Meditation:
- Lie Down Comfortably: Lie on your back with your arms by your sides and your legs uncrossed.

- Focus on Each Body Part: Starting from your toes, slowly bring your attention to each part of your body, noticing any sensations, tension, or pain. Move upwards towards your head.

- Breathe into Discomfort: If you notice tension or pain in your back, focus on that area and breathe deeply into it, imagining the breath bringing relief and relaxation.

- Practice Regularly: Perform this scan for 10-20 minutes, 1-2 times a day.

Both deep breathing exercises and meditation are simple yet powerful tools that can significantly reduce stress and muscle tension, thereby helping to relieve back pain. Regular practice will yield the best results, so it's beneficial to incorporate these techniques into your daily routine.

HOW OFTEN SHOULD I TAKE BREAKS TO RELAX AND RELIEVE STRESS WHEN DEALING WITH ACUTE BACK PAIN?

When dealing with acute back pain, taking regular breaks to relax and relieve stress is crucial for both pain management and overall recovery. Here's a guideline on how often and how to structure these breaks:

Frequency of Breaks:

- Every 20-30 Minutes: If you're engaged in an activity that involves sitting, standing, or repetitive movements (e.g., working at a desk or driving), aim to take a break every 20-30 minutes. Prolonged periods in the same position can increase muscle tension and exacerbate back pain.

- 5-Minute Breaks: During these breaks, spend at least 5 minutes moving around, stretching, or performing deep breathing exercises. This helps reduce muscle stiffness, improve circulation, and relieve stress.

- Hourly Breaks: In addition to shorter breaks every 20-30 minutes, take a slightly longer break of about 10-15 minutes every hour. Use this time to do a more thorough stretch, engage in relaxation exercises, or change your environment.

- Scheduled Relaxation Sessions: Incorporate scheduled relaxation or stress-relief sessions into your day. For example, practice deep breathing exercises, meditation, or progressive muscle relaxation for 10-20 minutes 2-3 times a day, especially during high-stress periods or when your back pain is more pronounced.

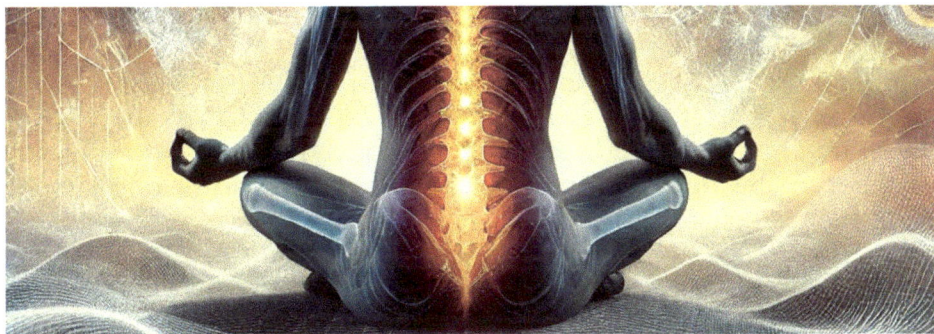

What to Do During Breaks:

- Stretching: Focus on gentle stretches that target the back, neck, and shoulders. Examples include the Cat-Cow stretch, seated forward bend, or gentle spinal twists.

- Movement: Engage in light movement like walking, marching in place, or doing simple exercises like shoulder rolls or ankle circles. Movement helps reduce stiffness and promote blood flow to your back muscles.

- Deep Breathing: Take a few minutes to practice deep breathing exercises. This can help reduce muscle tension and lower your stress levels.

- Posture Check: Use your breaks to check and adjust your posture. Ensure your sitting or standing posture is ergonomically correct, with proper support for your back.

- Mindful Relaxation: Close your eyes and focus on relaxing your muscles, starting from your feet, and working your way up to your head. This practice helps release tension from the body and mind.

Why Frequent Breaks Are Important:

- Prevents Muscle Fatigue: Regular breaks help prevent the muscles in your back from becoming overly fatigued, which can worsen pain.

- Reduces Stress Buildup: Frequent breaks allow you to manage stress levels throughout the day, preventing stress from accumulating and exacerbating your back pain.

- Promotes Healing: Taking breaks and relaxing helps promote circulation, reduce inflammation, and facilitate the healing process in your back.

By incorporating regular breaks and relaxation practices into your day, you can better manage acute back pain, reduce stress, and support your overall recovery.

CAN LISTENING TO MUSIC OR USING AROMATHERAPY HELP REDUCE STRESS AND ALLEVIATE MY BACK PAIN?

Both listening to music and using aromatherapy can help reduce stress and potentially alleviate back pain. These complementary therapies work by promoting relaxation, improving mood, and reducing the perception of pain.

How Music Can Help Reduce Stress and Alleviate Back Pain:
- Reduces Stress and Anxiety: Listening to calming music can lower stress levels by decreasing the production of cortisol, the stress hormone. It can also reduce anxiety, which is often linked to increased muscle tension and pain.

- Distracts from Pain: Music can serve as a distraction, diverting your attention away from the pain and making it feel less intense. This is particularly effective with music that you enjoy or find soothing.

- Promotes Relaxation: Certain types of music, especially those with slow tempos and low tones, can induce a state of relaxation, helping to release muscle tension in the back.

- Enhances Mood: Music can elevate your mood, which in turn can affect how you perceive and cope with pain. A positive mood can make pain feel less overwhelming.

How to Use Music for Back Pain Relief:
- Create a Playlist: Choose a playlist of calming or soothing music, such as classical, ambient, or nature sounds, that you can listen to during stressful times or when your back pain flares up.

- Use During Breaks: Listen to music during your regular breaks to help you relax and reset.

- Before Sleep: Listening to calming music before bed can improve sleep quality, which is essential for recovery and pain management.

How Aromatherapy Can Help Reduce Stress and Alleviate Back Pain:
- Reduces Stress and Promotes Relaxation: Certain essential oils, like lavender, chamomile, and ylang-ylang, are known for their calming

effects. Inhaling these scents can help reduce stress and anxiety, which can indirectly alleviate back pain.

- Reduces Muscle Tension: Aromatherapy can help relax tense muscles when used in conjunction with massage or applied topically in diluted forms. This can be particularly beneficial for back pain.

- Improves Sleep: Aromatherapy can improve sleep quality by creating a relaxing environment. Better sleep can enhance the body's ability to heal and reduce pain.

How to Use Aromatherapy for Back Pain Relief:
- Diffusion: Use an essential oil diffuser to disperse calming scents throughout your environment. Lavender, eucalyptus, and peppermint are popular choices for relaxation and pain relief.

- Topical Application: Dilute essential oils with a carrier oil (like coconut or jojoba oil) and apply them to the skin. For back pain, you can massage the diluted oil directly onto the affected area. Be cautious with the concentration and avoid applying oils directly to broken or irritated skin.

- Aromatherapy Baths: Add a few drops of essential oils to a warm bath. The combination of warm water and soothing scents can help relax muscles and reduce pain.

Combining Music and Aromatherapy:
You can enhance the stress-relief and pain management effects by combining music and aromatherapy. For example, you could play calming music while diffusing essential oils during a relaxation session or use both before bed to improve sleep quality.

Both music and aromatherapy are simple, non-invasive methods that can complement other treatments for back pain. The influence they have on the hormonal system and the effect that this has on our brain is beneficial to pain management. By reducing stress and promoting relaxation, these therapies can make a noticeable difference in how you experience and manage back pain. Incorporating them into your daily routine, especially during high-stress periods or pain flare-ups, can be particularly beneficial.

IS IT SAFE TO USE HEAT THERAPY OR TAKE WARM BATHS FOR STRESS RELIEF WHEN I HAVE ACUTE BACK PAIN?

It is safe to use heat therapy or take warm baths for stress relief when you have acute back pain, but there are some important considerations to keep in mind to ensure safety and effectiveness.

Benefits of Heat Therapy for Acute Back Pain:
- Reduces Muscle Tension: Heat helps to relax tight muscles, which can reduce pain and stiffness in the back. This relaxation effect also aids in stress relief.

- Improves Blood Circulation: Applying heat increases blood flow to the affected area, promoting healing by bringing more oxygen and nutrients to the tissues.

- Enhances Flexibility: Heat can improve the elasticity of muscles and soft tissues, making it easier to move and stretch, which can be beneficial during the acute phase of back pain.

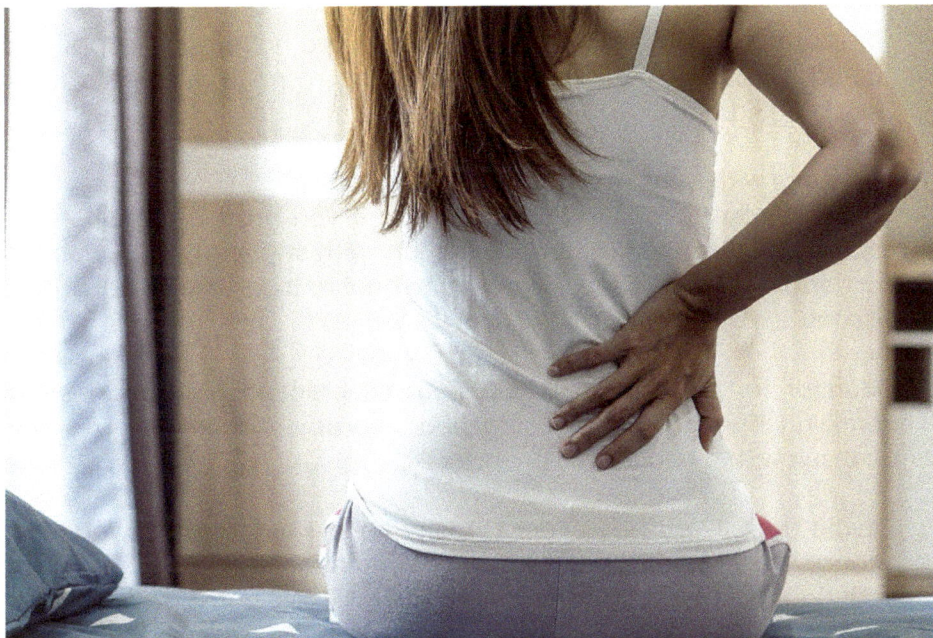

How to Safely Use Heat Therapy:
Heating Pads or Hot Packs:
- Use a Moderate Temperature: Ensure the heating pad or hot pack is warm, not hot, to avoid burns. It should feel comfortable against your skin.

- Limit Time: Apply heat for 15-20 minutes at a time. Overuse can lead to burns or increased inflammation.

- Use a Barrier: Place a cloth or towel between the heat source and your skin to prevent direct contact, which can cause burns.

Warm Baths:
- Moderate Temperature: Keep the water warm, not too hot. A temperature around 92-100°F (33-38°C) is generally safe and effective.

- Time Limit: Limit your bath to 20-30 minutes to avoid overheating or causing additional inflammation.

- Add Epsom Salts: Consider adding Epsom salts to your bath. The magnesium in Epsom salts can help relax muscles and reduce pain.

- Be Cautious Getting in and Out: Ensure you have good support to avoid slipping, as acute back pain can make movements more challenging.

Precautions with Heat Therapy and Warm Baths:
- Avoid If You Have Certain Conditions: If you have a condition like acute inflammation (e.g., a fresh injury with swelling), open wounds, or certain skin conditions, avoid using heat as it can exacerbate these issues.

- Monitor for Discomfort: If you notice increased pain, redness, or swelling during or after using heat therapy, discontinue use and consult with a healthcare provider.

- Avoid Heat if You Have Poor Circulation or Neuropathy: If you have conditions that impair sensation or circulation, such as diabetes, be cautious with heat therapy as you may not feel burns or damage to the skin.

Heat therapy and warm baths can be safe and effective methods for relieving stress and managing acute back pain when used appropriately. They can help reduce muscle tension, improve circulation, and promote relaxation, all of which contribute to pain relief. However, it's important to use these methods carefully, avoiding excessive heat and prolonged exposure, and to consult with a healthcare provider if you have any underlying health concerns or if your pain persists or worsens.

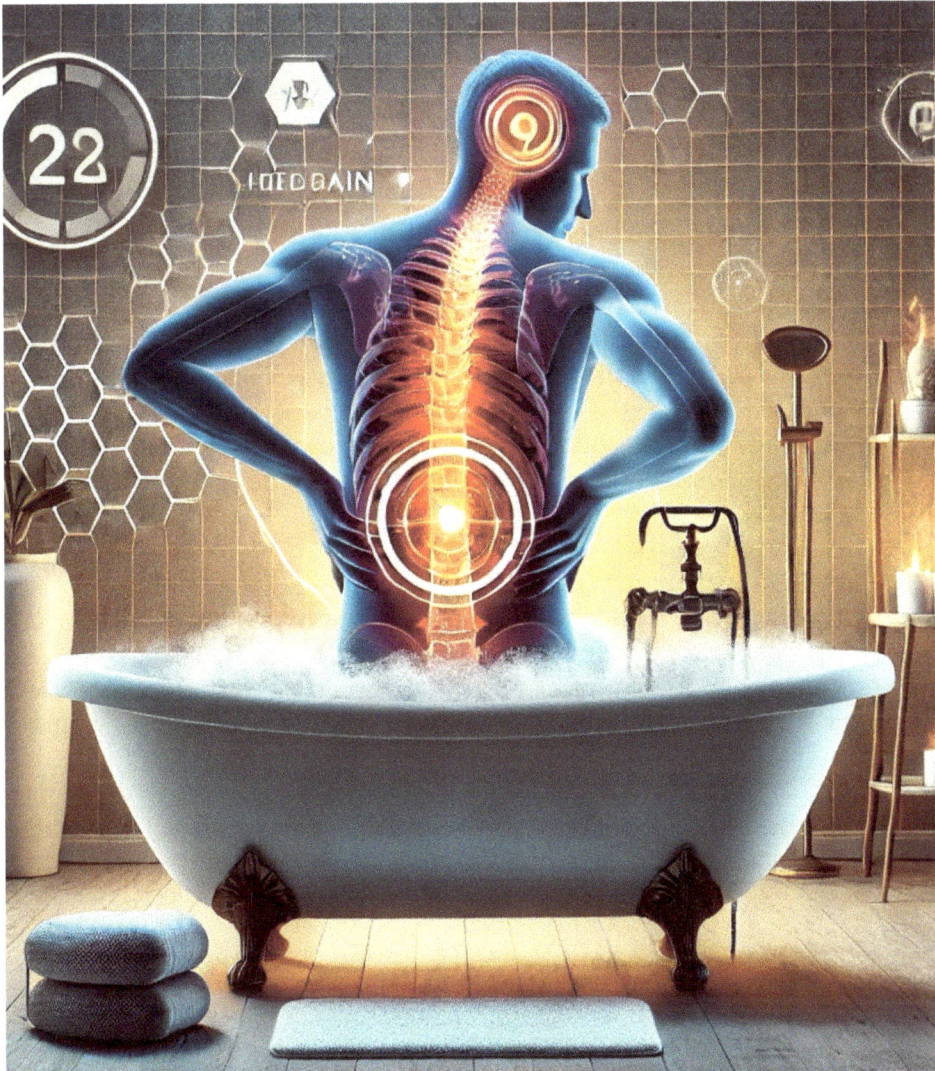

HOW CAN I MANAGE MY DAILY RESPONSIBILITIES AND STRESS WITHOUT WORSENING MY BACK PAIN?

Managing daily responsibilities and stress without worsening your back pain requires a combination of practical strategies and self-care techniques. Here are some tips to help you balance your responsibilities while protecting your back:

Prioritise and Delegate Tasks:
- Prioritise Important Tasks: Focus on the most essential tasks first. Break them down into manageable steps to avoid feeling overwhelmed.

- Delegate When Possible: Don't hesitate to ask for help with tasks that may strain your back. This can include household chores, lifting heavy objects, or even work-related responsibilities.

Incorporate Movement and Breaks:
- Frequent Breaks: As mentioned earlier, take short breaks every 20-30 minutes if you're sitting or standing for extended periods. Use these breaks to stretch, walk around, or do light exercises.

- Stretching Exercises: Incorporate gentle stretches for your back, neck, and shoulders throughout the day to reduce tension and improve flexibility.

Ergonomic Adjustments:
- Optimise Your Workstation: Ensure your chair, desk, and computer setup are ergonomically designed to support good posture and reduce strain on your back. Your feet should be flat on the floor, with your knees at a 90-degree angle and your computer screen at eye level.

- Use Supportive Footwear: If you're on your feet a lot, wear supportive shoes with good cushioning to reduce strain on your back.

Time Management and Stress Reduction:
- Plan Your Day: Create a realistic daily schedule that allows for breaks and relaxation. Avoid overcommitting yourself, which can lead to stress and worsen your back pain.

- Mindfulness and Relaxation Techniques: Incorporate stress-relief practices like mindfulness meditation, deep breathing, or yoga into your daily routine to help manage stress and reduce muscle tension.

Practice Good Body Mechanics:
- Lifting Techniques: When lifting objects, bend at your knees and hips, not your back. Keep the object close to your body and avoid twisting while lifting.

- Posture Awareness: Maintain good posture throughout the day, whether sitting, standing, or walking. Avoid slouching or hunching over, as this can increase back strain.

Use Assistive Devices:
- Back Supports: Consider using a lumbar roll or cushion when sitting to maintain the natural curve of your spine.

- Adaptive Tools: Use tools like grabbers or long-handled devices to avoid bending or reaching excessively.

Stay Active, but Know Your Limits:
- Gentle Exercise: Engage in low-impact exercises like walking, swimming, or cycling to keep your muscles strong and flexible without overexerting your back.

- Listen to Your Body: Pay attention to your body's signals. If an activity causes pain, stop and reassess how you're doing it. Rest when needed to avoid aggravating your back pain

Stay Active, but Know Your Limits:
- Nutrition and Hydration: Eat a balanced diet and stay hydrated. Proper nutrition supports overall health and healing.

- Sleep: Ensure you get enough rest each night, as sleep is essential for recovery and stress management. Use a supportive mattress and pillows that maintain spinal alignment.

Communicate and Set Boundaries:
- Set Realistic Expectations: Communicate your limitations to others, whether at work or home, to set realistic expectations and avoid overburdening yourself.

- Say No When Necessary: It's important to recognise when you need to say no to additional responsibilities that could exacerbate your condition.

Communicate and Set Boundaries:
- Physical Therapy: If your back pain persists or worsens, consider working with a physical therapist who can design a specific exercise program to strengthen your back and improve your posture.

- Mental Health Support: If stress is significantly impacting your life, speaking with a counsellor or therapist can provide strategies to manage stress more effectively.

By incorporating these strategies into your daily routine, you can manage your responsibilities and stress more effectively without worsening your back pain. Balancing self-care with your duties is key to maintaining both your health and productivity.

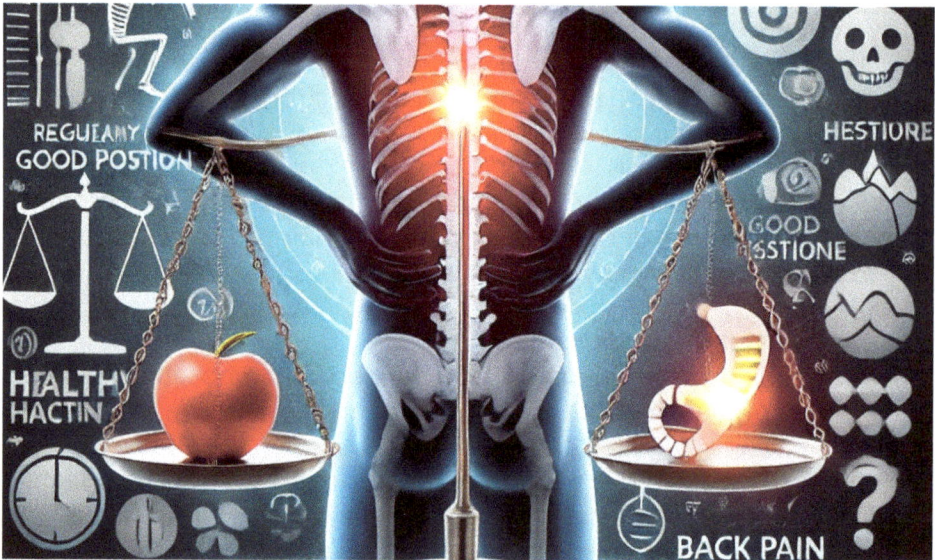

ARE THERE ANY GENTLE PHYSICAL ACTIVITIES, LIKE YOGA OR TAI CHI, WHICH CAN HELP WITH BOTH STRESS AND BACK PAIN MANAGEMENT?

Gentle physical activities like yoga and tai chi are highly effective for managing both stress and back pain. These practices focus on slow, controlled movements, breathing techniques, and mindfulness, making them ideal for improving flexibility, strength, and relaxation.

Yoga:

How It Helps:
- Improves Flexibility and Strength: Yoga stretches and strengthens the muscles, particularly those in the back, core, and legs. This can help alleviate back pain by improving posture and reducing muscle imbalances.

- Reduces Stress: The mindfulness and deep breathing techniques in yoga help reduce stress, which in turn can decrease muscle tension and pain perception.

- Enhances Body Awareness: Yoga increases your awareness of body alignment and movement patterns, helping you identify and correct habits that might contribute to back pain.

Gentle Yoga Poses for Back Pain:
- Child's Pose: A gentle stretch for the lower back.

- Cat-Cow Stretch: Improves flexibility in the spine and relieves tension in the back.

- Supine Twist: Stretches the spine and helps relieve lower back pain.

- Downward-Facing Dog: Stretches the back, hamstrings, and calves, promoting overall flexibility.

How to Practice:
- Start with a beginner or gentle yoga class, either in-person or online, focusing on back pain relief.

- Practice 2-3 times a week, gradually increasing the duration as your flexibility and strength improve.

Tai Chi:

How It Helps:
- Promotes Relaxation: Tai chi is often described as "meditation in motion," and its slow, flowing movements can help reduce stress and promote a calm, centred mind.

- Improves Balance and Posture: Tai chi enhances body awareness, balance, and posture, which are crucial for preventing and managing back pain.

- Strengthens Muscles: The controlled movements in tai chi strengthen the muscles of the legs, core, and back without putting too much strain on the body.

Basic Tai Chi Movements:
- Commencement: A gentle opening movement that promotes relaxation and prepares the body for more dynamic movements.

- Parting the Wild Horse's Mane: A movement that involves shifting weight and moving the arms in a flowing, circular pattern, which helps with balance and coordination.

- Wave Hands Like Clouds: Involves slow, side-to-side movements that help improve flexibility and coordination in the upper body.

How to Practice:
- Look for a beginner tai chi class or follow an instructional video. Classes designed for older adults or beginners are often gentler and focus on movements that are easier on the back.

- Practice tai chi regularly, aiming for 20-30 minutes per session, 2-3 times a week.

Other Gentle Activities:

- Pilates: Focuses on core strength, flexibility, and posture. Pilates can be particularly beneficial for strengthening the muscles that support the back.

- Walking: A simple, low-impact exercise that helps improve circulation, reduce stiffness, and relieve stress.

Tips for Getting Started:

- Start Slowly: If you're new to these activities, begin with short sessions and gradually increase the duration and intensity as your body adapts.

- Listen to Your Body: Pay attention to how your body feels during and after these activities. Avoid movements that cause pain and modify poses or exercises as needed.

- Consistency is Key: Regular practice is essential for achieving the benefits of these activities. Consistency will help you build strength, flexibility, and stress resilience over time.

Incorporating yoga, tai chi, or similar gentle activities into your routine can provide significant benefits for both stress and back pain management, promoting overall well-being and helping you maintain a healthy balance in your life.

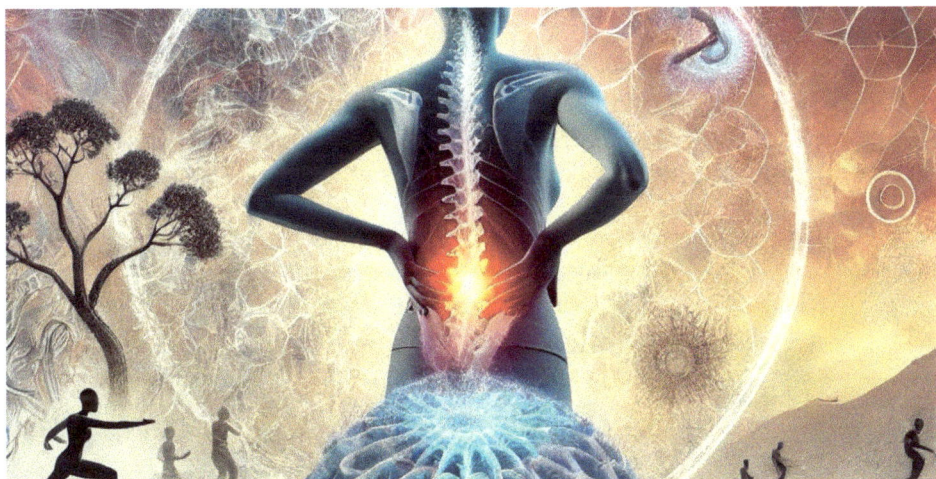

SHOULD I CONSIDER SPEAKING WITH A THERAPIST OR COUNSELLOR TO HELP MANAGE STRESS RELATED TO MY BACK PAIN?

Speaking with a therapist or counsellor can be a remarkably effective approach to managing stress related to your back pain. Chronic or acute back pain can be emotionally and mentally taxing and addressing the psychological aspects of pain can significantly improve your overall well-being and pain management strategies.

How a Psychotherapist or Counsellor Can Help:

Addressing the Emotional Impact of Pain:
- Coping with Chronic Pain: Chronic back pain can lead to feelings of frustration, anxiety, and depression. A therapist can help you process these emotions and develop healthier coping mechanisms.

- Reducing Pain Catastrophising: Pain catastrophising is when you anticipate or focus on pain excessively, which can make it feel worse. Cognitive Behavioural Therapy (CBT) is particularly effective in helping reduce these negative thought patterns.

Stress Management:
- Developing Stress-Relief Strategies: A therapist can work with you to identify the sources of stress related to your pain and teach you strategies to manage it, such as relaxation techniques, mindfulness, or guided imagery.

- Improving Sleep and Rest: Chronic pain often disrupts sleep, which can exacerbate stress. Therapy can help you develop better sleep habits and address any anxiety or stress that might be affecting your rest.

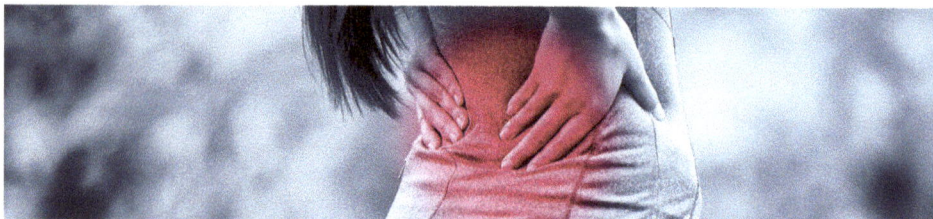

Behavioural Changes:

- Encouraging Positive Lifestyle Changes: Therapists can help you make lifestyle changes that support pain management, such as incorporating regular physical activity, improving diet, and maintaining social connections.

- Setting Realistic Goals: A therapist can help you set achievable goals related to your health and daily activities, which can reduce the stress associated with feeling overwhelmed by your pain.

Support and Validation:

- Providing Emotional Support: Sometimes, just having someone to talk to about your pain and its impact on your life can be incredibly relieving. Therapists offer a non-judgmental space to express your feelings and frustrations.

- Enhancing Social Support: A counsellor can also guide you in strengthening your social support network, which is crucial for managing both stress and pain.

Pain Management Techniques:

- Mind-Body Approaches: Therapists can teach mind-body techniques, such as biofeedback or relaxation training, which can help you gain more control over your pain.

- Mindfulness-Based Stress Reduction (MBSR): This program combines mindfulness meditation and yoga to help manage pain and stress and is often recommended by therapists for chronic pain sufferers.

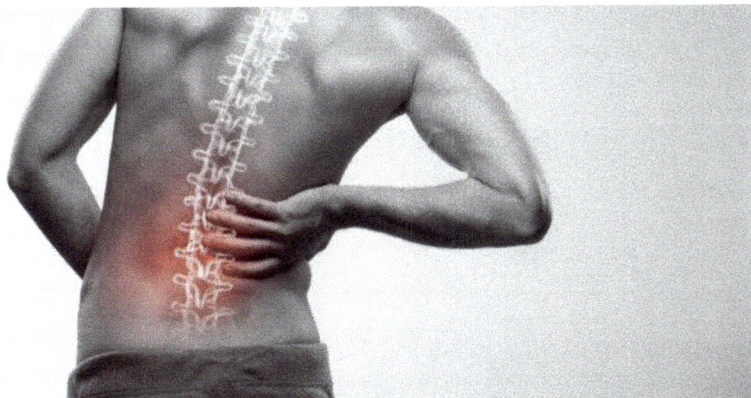

When to Consider Speaking with a Therapist:

- Persistent Stress or Anxiety: If your back pain is causing ongoing stress, anxiety, or depression that you're struggling to manage on your own, it's a good idea to seek professional help.

- Difficulty Coping: If you find it challenging to cope with the impact of your pain on your daily life, work, or relationships, a therapist can provide valuable support and tools.

- Worsening Pain Perception: If you notice that your pain feels more intense when you're stressed or anxious, therapy can help you address the psychological factors contributing to this.

How to Get Started:

- Consult Your Healthcare Provider: Talk to your doctor about a referral to a therapist or counsellor who specialises in pain management or chronic illness.

- Look for a Specialist: Consider finding a therapist with experience in treating patients with chronic pain, or someone who offers CBT, mindfulness, or other relevant therapies.

- Consider Online Therapy: If in-person sessions are difficult due to your back pain or other constraints, online therapy options are also available and can be effective.

In summary, speaking with a therapist or counsellor can be a valuable part of your back pain management plan, particularly if stress is exacerbating your condition. It can provide you with the emotional tools and strategies needed to manage both your pain and the stress that comes with it.

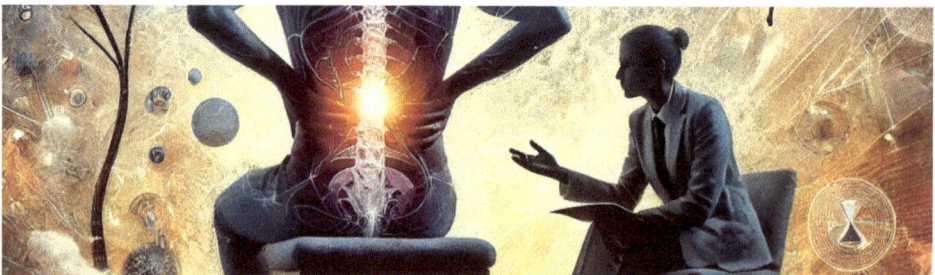

HOW TO BALANCE INTIMATE ACTIVITIES AND BACK PAIN

These questions highlight the relationship between stress and back pain, especially during the acute phase, and explore practical ways to manage stress to improve pain outcomes.

IS IT NECESSARY TO AVOID SEXUAL ACTIVITY DURING THE ACUTE PHASE OF MY BACK PAIN?

Whether or not to avoid sexual activity during the acute phase of back pain depends on several factors, including the severity of your pain, the specific nature of your back injury, and how your body responds to movement. Here are some considerations to help you make an informed decision:

Severity of Pain and Injury

Listen to Your Body: If engaging in sexual activity causes significant pain or discomfort, it may be best to avoid it until your back pain improves.

Type of Injury: Certain back injuries, like a herniated disc or muscle strain, may be aggravated by specific movements or positions. Understanding the nature of your injury can help you assess what activities to avoid.

Communication with Your Partner

Discuss Your Condition: Openly communicate with your partner about your pain and any limitations you may have. This can help you both adjust expectations and find positions or activities that are comfortable for you.

Experiment with Comfortable Positions: If you choose to engage in sexual activity, experimenting with positions that place less strain on your back, such as lying on your side or using pillows for support, may be helpful.

Impact on Recovery

Avoid Strain: If sexual activity exacerbates your pain or places strain on your back, it could delay your recovery. It's essential to avoid movements that might worsen your condition.

Consult Your Healthcare Provider: If you're unsure about the impact of sexual activity on your back pain, it's a good idea to discuss it with your healthcare provider. They can provide guidance based on your specific condition.

Alternative Intimacy

Explore Non-Physical Intimacy: If sexual activity is too painful, consider focusing on non-physical forms of intimacy, such as emotional connection, massage, or other forms of affectionate touch that do not strain your back.

Pain Management

Pre-Activity Preparation: If you decide to engage in sexual activity, taking steps to manage your pain beforehand, such as applying heat to your back or taking pain-relief medication (as advised by your doctor), might help.

Post-Activity Care: After sexual activity, consider using ice or heat, stretching, or practicing relaxation techniques to help manage any discomfort.

While it's not strictly necessary to avoid sexual activity during the acute phase of back pain, it's crucial to prioritise your comfort and recovery. If sexual activity exacerbates your pain, it may be best to wait until your back has healed more. Always listen to your body, communicate with your partner, and consider consulting your healthcare provider for personalised advice.

HOW CAN I TELL IF SEXUAL ACTIVITY IS SAFE OR IF IT MIGHT WORSEN MY BACK PAIN?

Determining whether sexual activity is safe or if it might worsen your back pain involves paying attention to your body's signals, understanding your specific condition, and being mindful of how different movements and positions affect you. Here's a guide to help you assess whether it's safe to engage in sexual activity:

Assess Your Current Pain Level:
- Baseline Pain: Consider how your back feels during daily activities. If you're experiencing significant pain during simple movements like bending, sitting, or walking, sexual activity might be too strenuous.

- Pain Response: If certain activities or positions cause sharp or intense pain, this could indicate that your back is not ready for sexual activity that requires similar movements.

Understand Your Injury or Condition:
- Type of Back Injury: Different back conditions may respond differently to physical activity. For example, a muscle strain might tolerate gentle movement, while a herniated disc might require more caution.

- Consultation with a Healthcare Provider: Discuss your condition with your doctor or physical therapist to understand which activities and movements should be avoided. They can offer advice on safe positions and movements based on your specific injury.

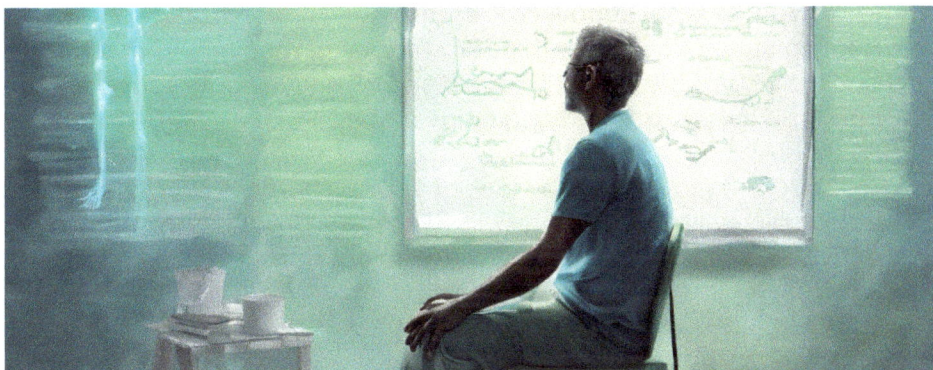

Experiment with Caution:
- Try Gentle Movements First: If you're uncertain, start with gentle, low-impact movements to see how your back responds. If you feel comfortable, you can gradually explore more activity.

- Stop If Pain Increases: If you notice an increase in pain during or after sexual activity, this is a sign that it may be exacerbating your condition. Stop immediately and try to identify which movements or positions caused discomfort.

Choose Positions Carefully:
- Positions that Reduce Strain: Consider positions that minimise strain on your back, such as lying on your side with your legs slightly bent or using pillows for support. Positions that require less movement or pressure on the spine are generally safer.

- Avoid High-Impact or Strenuous Positions: Positions that involve bending, twisting, or putting pressure on your back may increase the risk of pain. Avoid positions that are known to strain the lower back.

Use Pain as a Guide:
- Immediate Pain During Activity: If you feel sharp, shooting, or sudden pain during sexual activity, stop immediately. This is a clear sign that your back may not be ready for that level of activity.

- Delayed Pain: Pay attention to how your back feels in the hours and days following sexual activity. If you experience increased pain afterward, it may be a sign that you should avoid sexual activity until your back improves.

Consider Your Overall Recovery Progress:
- Healing Stage: If you're in the early stages of recovery from an acute back injury, it's often best to avoid sexual activity until your back has had time to heal and your pain has stabilised.

- Track Your Recovery: Keep track of your symptoms over time. If your back pain is steadily improving, you may gradually resume more activities, including sexual activity, with caution.

Communicate with Your Partner:
- Open Communication: Discuss your pain and any concerns with your partner. Together, you can explore what feels comfortable and safe for both of you.

- Take It Slow: Start slowly and adjust based on your comfort level. Be willing to stop if you feel any discomfort.

Use Supportive Measures:
- Pain Management: If approved by your healthcare provider, consider using heat therapy, stretching, or pain relief medication before sexual activity to reduce discomfort.

- Post-Activity Care: After sexual activity, use ice, heat, or gentle stretching to help alleviate any discomfort that may arise.

To determine if sexual activity is safe for you, listen to your body, consider your specific back condition, and proceed with caution. If sexual activity increases your pain or causes discomfort, it's best to wait until your back is in a better state of recovery. Consulting with a healthcare provider for personalised advice is also a wise approach.

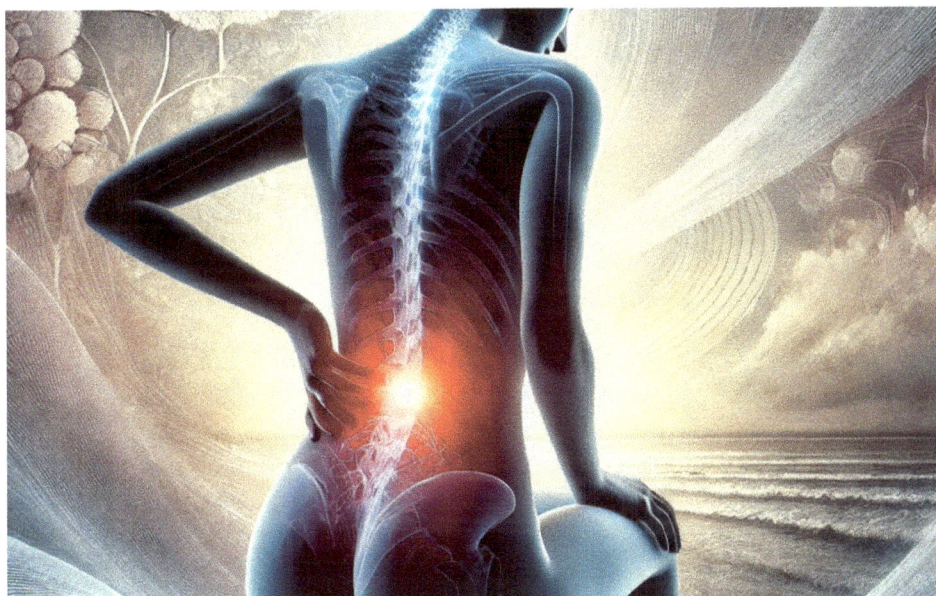

ARE THERE SPECIFIC POSITIONS OR MOVEMENTS I SHOULD AVOID IN THE ATTEMPT TO PREVENT AGGRAVATING MY BACK PAIN DURING SEX?

There are specific positions and movements you should avoid during sex to prevent aggravating your back pain. The key is to minimise strain on the back, especially the lower back, and to avoid positions that involve excessive bending, twisting, or pressure on the spine. Here are some guidelines.

Positions and Movements to Avoid:

Excessive Bending or Arching of the Back:
- Avoid Positions that Require Hyperextension: Positions where your back is excessively arched or hyperextended, such as lying on your stomach or positions that require a deep backbend, can put significant strain on the lumbar spine.

- Example to Avoid: Positions like "doggy style" (with the receiving partner on hands and knees) may cause excessive arching of the back, which can exacerbate lower back pain.

Twisting Movements:
- Avoid Twisting the Spine: Positions that require twisting or rotating your torso can strain the spine and aggravate back pain.

- Example to Avoid: Positions that involve turning the upper body in one direction while the lower body remains stationary, or any movement that involves a twist, should be avoided.

Unsupported, Upright Positions:
- Avoid Standing or Sitting Without Support: Positions that require standing, sitting, or kneeling without adequate back support can place a lot of pressure on the lower back.

- Example to Avoid: Unsupported standing or sitting positions, especially if they involve repetitive or thrusting movements, can be particularly challenging for those with back pain.

High-Impact or Strenuous Movements:
- Avoid Rapid or Forceful Movements: Fast, jerky, or forceful movements can jolt the spine and exacerbate back pain.

- Example to Avoid: Movements that involve significant impact or force, such as vigorous thrusting, should be avoided if they cause discomfort.

Positions and Movements that May Be Safer:

Side-Lying (Spooning) Position:
- How It Helps: Lying on your side with your legs slightly bent can keep the spine in a neutral position and reduce strain on the back.

- Adjustments: Placing a pillow between your knees can further alleviate pressure on the lower back.

Missionary Position with Support:
- How It Helps: If you're on your back, placing a pillow under your knees can help maintain the natural curve of the spine, reducing strain.

- Adjustments: The partner on top can control movement, allowing for slow and gentle actions that minimise strain.

Modified Woman-on-Top Position:
- How It Helps: If the partner with back pain is on top, they can control the depth and speed of movement, allowing for positions that are less stressful on the back.

- Adjustments: The partner on top can lean forward, placing less pressure on the lower back. Alternatively, leaning back slightly while supporting themselves with their hands can reduce strain.

Using Supportive Props:
- How It Helps: Pillows or wedges can be used to support the back and pelvis, keeping the spine in a more neutral and comfortable position.

- Adjustments: Experiment with different support placements to find what feels best for your back.

Tips for Managing Back Pain During Sex:

- Persistent Stress or Anxiety: If your back pain is causing ongoing stress, anxiety, or depression that you're struggling to manage on your o

Communicate with Your Partner:
Openly discuss your pain and any concerns you have. This helps both partners feel comfortable adjusting positions as needed.

Move Slowly and Gently:
Slow, controlled movements reduce the risk of jarring the spine or causing a muscle spasm.

Warm Up with Gentle Stretching:
Before engaging in sexual activity, try some gentle stretches to loosen up your back muscles. Simple stretches like cat-cow or child's pose can help.

Post-Activity Care:
After sex, consider applying heat or ice to your back, doing some light stretching, or using relaxation techniques to ease any tension or discomfort.

By avoiding positions and movements that place undue stress on your back and opting for safer alternatives, you can engage in sexual activity with reduced risk of aggravating your back pain. Always listen to your body, and don't hesitate to stop or adjust if you experience discomfort.

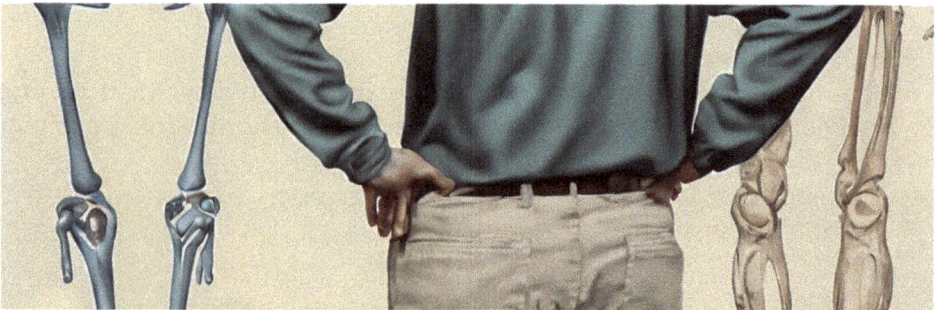

CAN SEXUAL ACTIVITY DELAY MY RECOVERY FROM ACUTE BACK PAIN, AND IF SO, HOW LONG SHOULD I WAIT?

Sexual activity can potentially delay recovery from acute back pain if it exacerbates the pain or involves movements that strain the injured area. However, whether it significantly impacts recovery depends on several factors, including the severity of your back pain, the specific nature of your injury, and how your body responds to physical activity.

How Sexual Activity Might Affect Recovery:

- Strain on the Back: Certain positions or movements during sexual activity can put stress on the muscles, ligaments, or discs in the back, potentially worsening the injury or delaying healing.

- Increased Pain: If sexual activity causes increased pain, it may lead to muscle spasms or further inflammation, which can prolong the recovery process.

- Interruption of Healing: The body needs time to heal from acute back pain, especially if it's due to a strain, sprain, or disc issue. Physical activities that overexert the back can interrupt this healing process.

When to Wait and How Long:

- Wait Until Pain Subsides: It's generally advisable to wait until the acute phase of your back pain has subsided before resuming sexual activity. This typically means waiting until your pain is manageable and does not flare up with light activities.

- Consult Your Healthcare Provider: Your doctor or physical therapist can give you personalised advice on when it might be safe to resume sexual activity based on the specifics of your condition. They can also suggest safe positions and movements.

- Listen to Your Body: If you experience discomfort, increased pain, or any signs of worsening back pain after sexual activity, it's a sign that your body might not be ready. In such cases, you should consider waiting longer.

General Guidelines for Waiting:

- Mild Back Pain: If your back pain is mild and you feel comfortable with daily activities, you might wait a few days to a week before trying sexual activity, taking care to avoid positions that strain your back.

- Moderate to Severe Pain: For more severe pain or injuries, it's usually better to wait at least 2-3 weeks or until you've made significant progress in your recovery. This is especially true if your pain increases with physical activity.

- Re-evaluation: If you're unsure, re-evaluate after a week or two of recovery. If your back feels significantly better and daily activities are no longer painful, you may consider resuming sexual activity cautiously.

Safe Resumption of Sexual Activity:

When you do resume sexual activity, start slowly, use positions that minimise back strain, and focus on gentle, controlled movements. Avoid any activities that cause discomfort and be prepared to stop if you feel any increase in pain.

In summary while sexual activity can potentially delay recovery from acute back pain if it aggravates your condition, the decision on when to resume it should be based on your level of pain, how your body responds to activity, and advice from your healthcare provider. Waiting until your back pain has improved and being cautious about the movements and positions you use can help ensure that you do not hinder your recovery.

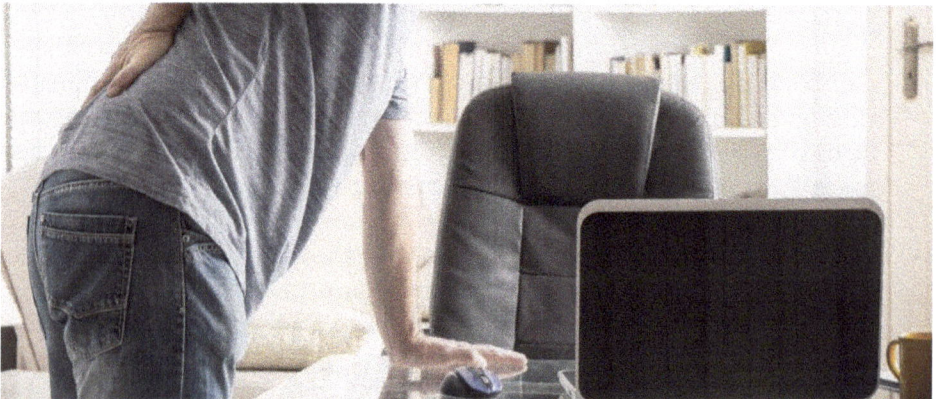

WHAT ARE SOME ALTERNATIVE WAYS TO MAINTAIN INTIMACY WITH MY PARTNER WHILE AVOIDING SEX DURING MY BACK PAIN FLARE-UP?

Maintaining intimacy with your partner during a back pain flare-up is important for your relationship, and there are many ways to stay connected and close without engaging in sexual activity. Here are some alternative ways to maintain intimacy:

Emotional Intimacy:
- Open Communication: Share your feelings, concerns, and experiences related to your back pain. This foster understanding and emotional closeness.

- Deep Conversations: Spend time talking about your dreams, memories, or anything meaningful to both of you. Deep, heartfelt conversations can strengthen your emotional bond.

Physical Affection:
- Cuddling: Cuddling can be a comforting way to maintain physical closeness. Find a position that is comfortable for your back, such as side-lying or using supportive pillows.

- Holding Hands: Simple gestures like holding hands while watching a movie or walking can reinforce your connection.

- Gentle Touch: Light massages, stroking, or simply touching each other's arms, face, or hair can be soothing and intimate.

Massage Therapy:
- Partner Massage: A gentle massage can help relieve muscle tension and pain. It's also a way to connect physically without putting strain on your back. Be sure to guide your partner on where and how to apply pressure based on what feels good for you.

- Aromatherapy Massage: Combine massage with aromatherapy by using essential oils like lavender or chamomile, which can enhance relaxation and intimacy.

Shared Activities:
- Watch a Movie or Series Together: Choose a comfortable spot and enjoy a movie or a series you both like. Sharing these moments can be very bonding.

- Cook a Meal Together: Preparing a meal together, even if it's something simple, can be a fun and intimate experience. If standing for prolonged periods is challenging, take breaks or delegate tasks.

- Read Aloud: Reading a book or poetry to each other can be an intimate way to spend time together, especially if it's something you both enjoy.

Create a Relaxing Environment:
- Take a Bath Together: If your back allows it, a warm bath can be soothing. Add Epsom salts or essential oils to create a spa-like experience. Be cautious about getting in and out of the bath, ensuring that your back is supported.

- Listen to Music: Share music that you both enjoy, slow dancing or just relaxing together while listening.

Engage in Mindfulness or Meditation Together:
- Mindfulness Exercises: Practice mindfulness or meditation together. This can involve deep breathing, guided meditation, or simply sitting quietly together in a peaceful environment.

- Yoga or Stretching: Gentle yoga or stretching exercises can be done together. These activities not only help with pain management but also create a sense of shared wellness.

Creative Expression:
- Write Letters or Notes: Writing love notes or letters to each other can be a deeply personal and intimate way to express your feelings, especially when physical activity is limited.

- Art or Craft Projects: Engaging in a creative project together, like painting or crafting, can be a fun way to bond while focusing on something positive and creative.

Plan for the Future:

- Plan a Future Date or Trip: Even if you can't be physically active right now, planning a future date, trip, or activity can be exciting and give you both something to look forward to.

- Set Relationship Goals: Discuss your goals as a couple, whether they are related to your relationship, health, or personal growth. This can reinforce your connection and mutual support.

Maintaining intimacy while avoiding sex during a back pain flare-up is entirely possible and can even deepen your relationship in new ways. By focusing on emotional connection, physical affection, and shared experiences, you can keep your bond strong and navigate this challenging time together.

IF I EXPERIENCE PAIN DURING SEX, SHOULD I STOP IMMEDIATELY, OR ARE THERE ADJUSTMENTS THAT CAN BE MADE TO CONTINUE SAFELY?

If you experience pain during sex, it's important to listen to your body. Whether you should stop immediately or make adjustments depends on the nature and intensity of the pain. Here's how to approach the situation:

Positions and Movements to Avoid:

Assess the Pain:
- Sharp or Intense Pain: If the pain is sharp, sudden, or severe, it's best to stop immediately. This type of pain could indicate that a movement or position is aggravating your back or causing further injury.

- Mild or Discomforting Pain: If the pain is mild or more of a discomfort, you might be able to continue with some adjustments, but it's important to proceed with caution.

Communicate with Your Partner:
- Pause and Discuss: Let your partner know that you're experiencing pain. Communication is key to finding a solution that works for both of you.

- Reevaluate Together: Decide together whether to continue with modifications or to stop altogether.

Make Adjustments:
- Change Positions: Try switching to a position that puts less strain on your back. For example, if a position involves arching your back or twisting, try one that allows your spine to stay more neutral, such as side-lying (spooning) or with added pillow support.

- Use Supportive Props: Adding pillows or cushions under your back, hips, or legs can help support your spine and reduce strain.

- Slow Down: Reducing the speed and intensity of movements can lessen the impact on your back. Gentle, controlled movements are less likely to cause pain

Monitor Your Pain:
- If Pain Persists: If the pain continues or worsens despite adjustments, it's important to stop and avoid further aggravation. Continuing through pain can lead to increased injury or prolonged recovery.

- If Pain Subsides: If making adjustments helps reduce or eliminate the pain, you may be able to continue more comfortably. However, remain mindful of your body and avoid pushing through discomfort.

Post-Activity Care:
- Rest and Recovery: After stopping or adjusting, take some time to rest. Apply heat or ice to your back if needed and consider doing some gentle stretches to relieve any lingering tension.

- Evaluate for Future: Reflect on what caused the pain and what adjustments worked. This can help you avoid similar issues in the future.

Seek Professional Advice:
- Consult a Healthcare Provider: If you frequently experience pain during sex or if the pain is severe, consult your doctor or a physical therapist. They can provide guidance on safe sexual positions and movements based on your specific back condition.

If you experience pain during sex, it's important to stop immediately if the pain is sharp or intense. For mild discomfort, you might try adjusting your position, pace, or use of support. However, if the pain persists or worsens, it's best to stop to prevent further injury. Always prioritise your health and well-being and seek professional advice if needed to find a comfortable and safe approach to intimacy.

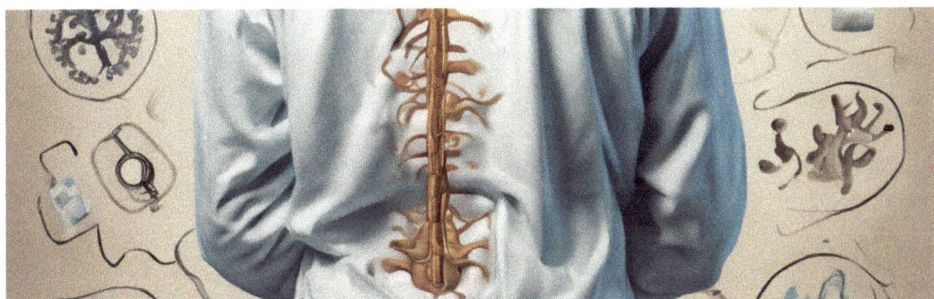

ARE THERE ANY GENTLE STRETCHES OR EXERCISES I CAN DO BEFORE SEX TO MINIMISE THE RISK OF BACK PAIN?

Performing gentle stretches or exercises before sex can help minimise the risk of back pain by warming up your muscles, increasing flexibility, and reducing tension in your back. Here are some recommended stretches and exercises that you can do to prepare your body and reduce the likelihood of discomfort:

Cat-Cow Stretch:

How It Helps: This stretch increases flexibility in the spine, promotes spinal mobility, and relieves tension in the back muscles.

How to Do It:

- Start on your hands and knees in a tabletop position, with your wrists aligned under your shoulders and your knees under your hips.

- Inhale as you arch your back, lifting your head and tailbone towards the ceiling (Cow Pose).

- Exhale as you round your back, tucking your chin to your chest and drawing your belly button towards your spine (Cat Pose).

- Repeat this flow for 5-10 cycles, moving slowly and gently.

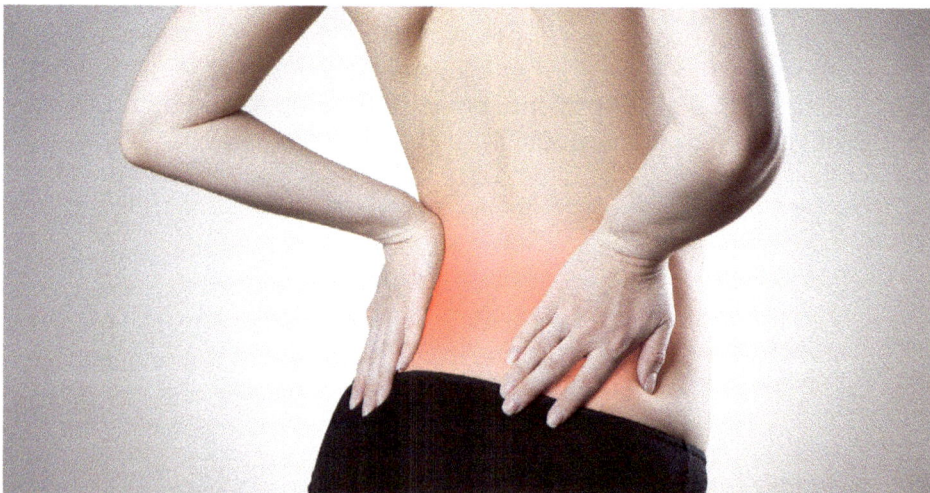

Child's Pose:

How It Helps: Child's Pose gently stretches the lower back, hips, and thighs, providing relief from tension and promoting relaxation.

How to Do It:
- Start on your hands and knees, then sit back onto your heels while extending your arms forward on the floor.

- Lower your chest towards the floor, resting your forehead on the mat.

- Hold the pose for 30 seconds to 1 minute, breathing deeply and allowing your back to relax.

Pelvic Tilts:

How It Helps: Pelvic tilts strengthen the lower abdominal muscles and promote mobility in the lower back, helping to alleviate stiffness.

How to Do It:
- Lie on your back with your knees bent and feet flat on the floor, hip-width apart.

- Flatten your lower back against the floor by tightening your abdominal muscles and tilting your pelvis slightly upward.

- Hold for a few seconds, then relax and return to the starting position.

- Repeat 10-15 times, moving slowly and focusing on the movement in your lower back.

Knee-to-Chest Stretch:

How It Helps: This stretch helps to release tension in the lower back and stretch the glutes and hamstrings.

How to Do It:
- Lie on your back with your knees bent and feet flat on the floor.

- Gently draw one knee towards your chest, holding it with both hands.

- Hold the stretch for 20-30 seconds, then switch to the other leg.

- For a deeper stretch, you can bring both knees to your chest at the same time.

Bridge Pose:

How It Helps: The Bridge Pose strengthens the glutes, hamstrings, and lower back, while also opening the hips and stretching the chest.

How to Do It:

- Lie on your back with your knees bent and feet flat on the floor, hip-width apart.

- Press your feet into the floor and lift your hips towards the ceiling, engaging your glutes and core.

- Hold the pose for 10-15 seconds, then slowly lower your hips back down to the floor.

- Repeat 5-10 times, focusing on controlled movements.

Seated Forward Bend:

How It Helps: This stretches targets the hamstrings, lower back, and hips, promoting flexibility and relieving tension.

How to Do It:

- Sit on the floor with your legs extended straight in front of you.

- Inhale and lengthen your spine, then exhale as you gently reach forward towards your feet, keeping your back straight.

- Hold the stretch for 20-30 seconds, breathing deeply, and avoid rounding your back.

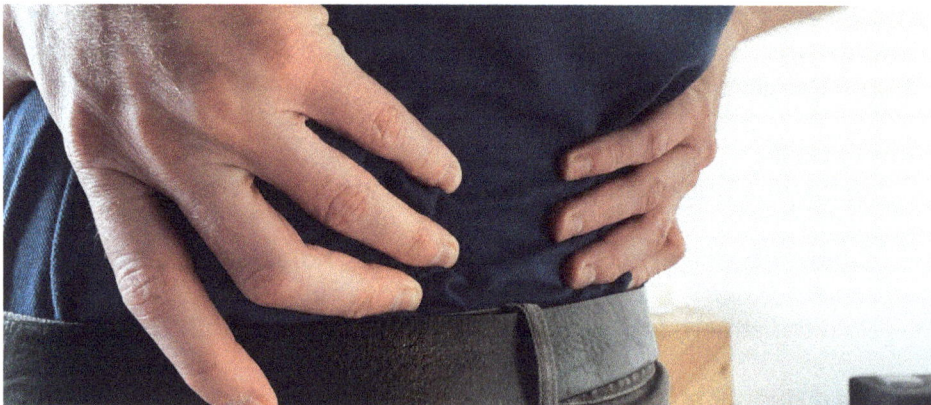

Spinal Twist (Supine Twist):

How It Helps: Twisting gently stretches the spine, hips, and shoulders, helping to release tension and improve mobility in the back.

How to Do It:

- Lie on your back with your knees bent and feet flat on the floor.

- Extend your arms out to the sides in a T-shape.

- Gently lower both knees to one side, keeping your shoulders flat on the floor.

- Hold the twist for 20-30 seconds, then switch to the other side.

STips for Performing Stretches and Exercises:

- Move Slowly and Gently: Avoid any sudden or forceful movements that could strain your back.

- Breathe Deeply: Focus on deep, steady breathing throughout each stretch to enhance relaxation and muscle release.

- Warm-Up: If you've been inactive, consider doing a light warm-up (like walking) before stretching to get your blood flowing and muscles warmed up.

If you incorporate these gentle stretches and exercises into your routine before engaging in sexual activity you can help prepare your body, reduce muscle tension, and minimise the risk of back pain. Always listen to your body and avoid pushing through any discomfort during these movements.

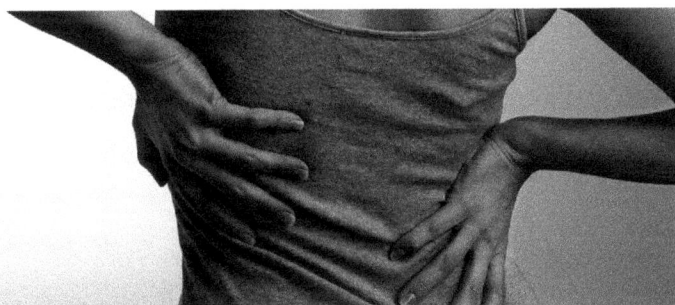

HOW CAN I COMMUNICATE WITH MY PARTNER ABOUT THE NEED TO AVOID OR MODIFY SEXUAL ACTIVITY DUE TO MY BACK PAIN?

Communicating with your partner about the need to avoid or modify sexual activity due to back pain can be a sensitive topic, but it's essential for maintaining both your physical health and the health of your relationship. Here's how to approach the conversation:

Choose the Right Time and Place:
- Private and Comfortable Setting: Have the conversation in a private, relaxed environment where you both feel comfortable.

- Avoid High-Stress Moments: Choose a time when neither of you is stressed or in a rush. Avoid bringing it up during or immediately after intimacy to prevent any feelings of rejection.

Be Honest and Direct:
- Explain Your Condition: Clearly explain your back pain, its impact on your daily life, and how it affects your ability to engage in sexual activity. Be open about what you're experiencing physically.

- Use "I" Statements: Frame your concerns using "I" statements to express how you feel without making your partner feel blamed. For example, "I'm feeling a lot of discomfort in my back right now, and I'm worried that certain activities might make it worse."

Express Your Need for Support:
- Ask for Understanding: Let your partner know that you need their understanding and support during this time. Emphasise that your goal is to protect your health and ensure a positive experience for both of you.

- Reassure Your Partner: Reassure your partner that your desire for intimacy hasn't changed, but that you need to find ways to be close without causing pain.

Suggest Alternatives:
- Discuss Modifications: Talk about modifying sexual activity to make it more comfortable. This could include trying different positions, slowing down the pace, or using pillows for support.

- Explore Other Forms of Intimacy: Suggest other ways to maintain intimacy, such as cuddling, massage, or spending quality time together. Let your partner know that closeness is still important to you.

Invite Collaboration:
- Ask for Their Input: Encourage your partner to share their thoughts and feelings about the situation. Ask for their input on what might work for both of you.

- Problem-Solve Together: Work together to find solutions that allow you to be intimate without causing pain. This might include experimenting with different activities or adjusting your approach to intimacy.

Keep the Conversation Ongoing:
- Check-In Regularly: Make it a point to check in with each other regularly about how you're both feeling, especially as your back pain evolves or improves.

- Be Open to Change: Be willing to revisit the conversation as needed, adjusting your approach as your condition changes.

Express Gratitude and Reassurance:
- Thank Your Partner: Acknowledge and appreciate your partner's understanding and support. Expressing gratitude can help strengthen your bond.

- Reaffirm Your Connection: Reaffirm your emotional and physical connection, and let your partner know that your desire for intimacy hasn't diminished, even if the way you express it needs to be adjusted temporarily.

Seek Professional Advice Together:
- Consider Counselling: If you're finding it difficult to communicate about this issue or if it's causing tension in your relationship, consider seeking couples counselling. A therapist can help facilitate the conversation and provide strategies for maintaining intimacy.

Example of How to Start the Conversation:

"Hey, I've been meaning to talk to you about something important. Lately, my back pain has been making certain activities very uncomfortable, and I'm worried that pushing through it could make things worse. I love being close to you, and I want to make sure we find ways to stay connected without causing more pain. Can we talk about how we can adjust things for now?"

In summary an effective communication about your back pain and its impact on your sexual activity is crucial for maintaining a healthy and supportive relationship. By being honest, expressing your needs, and working together to find alternatives, you can ensure that both you and your partner feel understood and connected, even during challenging times.

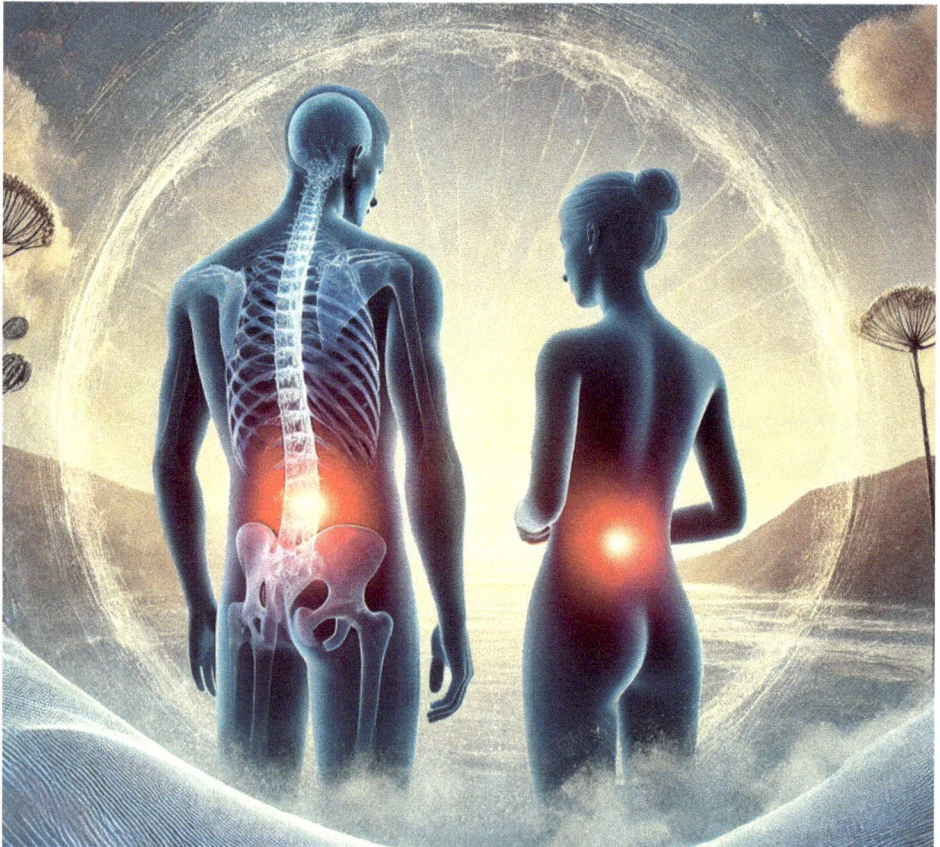

IS IT BETTER TO AVOID SEX ALTOGETHER DURING ACUTE BACK PAIN, OR ARE THERE SAFER WAYS TO ENGAGE IN SEXUAL ACTIVITY?

Whether to avoid sex altogether during acute back pain or find safer ways to engage in sexual activity depends on the severity of your pain, your personal comfort level, and your ability to modify activities to avoid aggravating your condition. Here's a guide to help you make an informed decision:

Evaluate Your Pain and Condition:
- Severity of Pain: If your pain is severe, constant, or worsens with movement, it may be best to avoid sexual activity until your condition improves.

- Type of Back Injury: Certain injuries, like a herniated disc or severe muscle strain, may require more caution and rest, making it advisable to avoid sex until you've healed.

Listen to Your Body:
- Pain as a Guide: Your body will usually give you clear signals if something isn't right. If sexual activity causes or increases pain, it's important to stop and reassess.

- Comfort Levels: If you feel uncomfortable or are concerned about worsening your condition, it may be better to focus on rest and recovery.

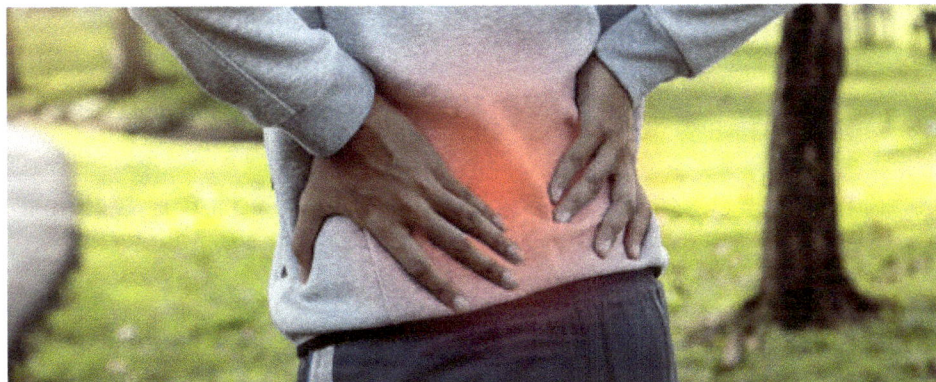

Consider Modifications for Safer Engagement:

If you decide to engage in sexual activity despite having acute back pain, here are some strategies to make it safer:

- Choose Gentle Positions: Opt for positions that minimise strain on the back, such as side-lying (spooning) or positions where you can maintain a neutral spine. Avoid positions that require arching, twisting, or putting pressure on your back.

- Use Supportive Props: Pillows, cushions, or wedges can help support your body and reduce strain on your back. For example, placing a pillow under your knees while lying on your back can help maintain spinal alignment.

- Slow and Controlled Movements: Engage in slow, gentle movements rather than fast or vigorous activity. This reduces the risk of jolting or straining your back.

- Communicate with Your Partner: Make sure your partner is aware of your condition and is willing to adjust their movements and expectations. Open communication is key to ensuring both partners feel comfortable and supported.

Focus on Non-Sexual Intimacy:

If you decide to avoid sexual activity, you can maintain intimacy in other ways:

- Physical Affection: Cuddling, holding hands, or giving each other massages are great ways to stay connected physically without putting strain on your back.

- Emotional Connection: Spend time together doing activities that promote emotional intimacy, such as talking, watching a movie, or sharing a hobby.

- Plan for the Future: If you're temporarily abstaining from sex, plan for when you can resume it safely. This anticipation can help maintain a positive connection with your partner.

Consult Your Healthcare Provider:

If you're unsure whether sexual activity is safe for you, consult your doctor or physical therapist. They can provide specific advice based on your own condition and suggest modifications that could make sex safer for you.

It has to be noted that there's no one-size-fits-all answer to whether you should avoid sex during acute back pain. If your pain is severe or worsens with movement, it may be better to rest and focus on recovery. However, if you feel up to it and can make the necessary adjustments, there are safer ways to engage in sexual activity without aggravating your condition. The most important thing is to listen to your body, communicate with your partner, and prioritise your health and comfort.

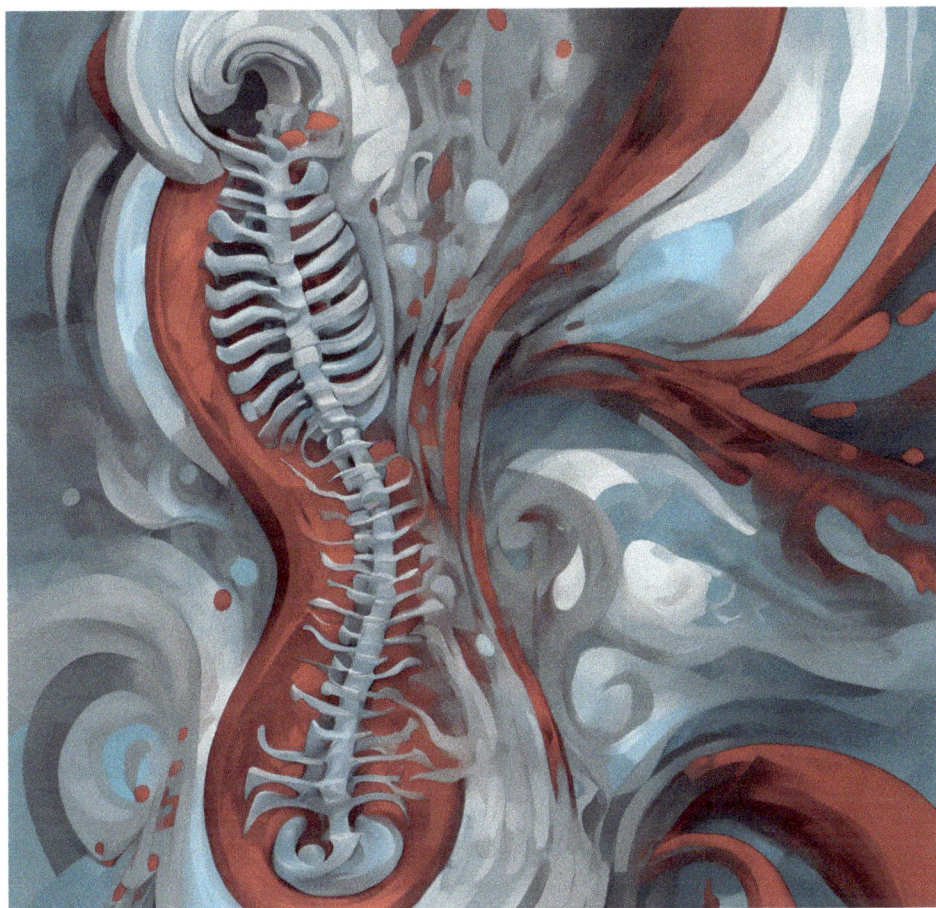

WHEN IS IT SAFE TO RESUME SEXUAL ACTIVITY AFTER EXPERIENCING AN ACUTE BACK PAIN EPISODE, AND WHAT SIGNS SHOULD I LOOK FOR TO KNOW IT'S OKAY?

Resuming sexual activity after experiencing an acute back pain episode should be approached with caution and experimentation. The timing depends on the severity of your pain, the nature of your injury, and how well your body has responded to rest and treatment. Here's a guide to help you determine when it might be safe to resume sexual activity and what signs to look for:

Signs That It May Be Safe to Resume Sexual Activity:
- Significant Pain Reduction: You should experience a noticeable reduction in pain, both in intensity and frequency. If your back pain has decreased significantly and you can perform daily activities without discomfort, it may be a sign that your body is ready.

- Improved Mobility: Your range of motion should be close to normal, with minimal stiffness or discomfort. You should be able to move, bend, and twist without sharp pain.

- Ability to Perform Light Physical Activity: If you can engage in light physical activities, such as walking, gentle stretching, or low-impact exercises, without triggering back pain, this indicates that your back is healing and might tolerate more activity.

- No Pain with Routine Movements: Everyday movements, like sitting, standing, or getting in and out of bed, should be pain-free. This suggests that your back can handle more dynamic movements.

- Stable Condition Over Time: Your back should feel stable and pain-free over several days or weeks, without any flare-ups or setbacks.

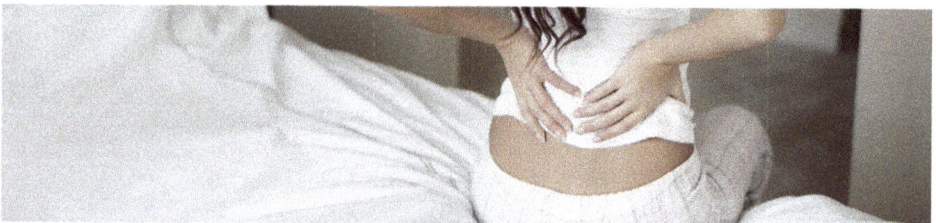

Precautions Before Resuming Sexual Activity:
- Consult with Your Healthcare Provider: If you're unsure, it's always a good idea to check with your doctor or physical therapist before resuming sexual activity. They can assess your recovery and provide specific advice based on your condition.

- Start Slowly and Gently: When you first resume sexual activity, start with gentle, low-impact positions that minimise strain on your back. Avoid any positions or movements that require significant twisting, arching, or bending of your spine.

- Use Supportive Props: Pillows and cushions can help support your back and reduce strain during sexual activity. Experiment with different placements to find what feels most comfortable.

- Communicate with Your Partner: Let your partner know that you're recovering and may need to take things slow. Open communication ensures that both partners are comfortable and that any adjustments can be made as needed.

Signs That You Should Continue to Wait:
- Persistent Pain or Discomfort: If you still experience pain during daily activities or specific movements, it's best to continue resting and avoid sexual activity.

- Pain with Certain Movements: If bending, twisting, or lifting causes pain, your back may not be ready for the dynamic movements involved in sexual activity.

- Flare-Ups: If your back pain flares up after certain activities or after trying to resume sexual activity, it's a clear sign that your body needs more time to heal.

- Feeling of Instability: If your back feels unstable, weak, or prone to "giving out," it's important to avoid sexual activity until you've regained strength and stability.

Monitoring Your Body's Response:

- After Activity Check: Pay attention to how your back feels after resuming sexual activity. If you experience any pain or discomfort during or after, stop and give your body more time to heal before trying again.

- Gradual Progression: Resume sexual activity gradually. Start with short sessions and gentle positions, and slowly increase as your comfort level and back condition improve.

It's safe to resume sexual activity after an acute back pain episode when you have significant pain reduction, improved mobility, and can perform daily activities without discomfort. Always listen to your body, and if you have any doubts, consult your healthcare provider. By taking it slow and being mindful of your body's signals, you can ensure that you resume sexual activity safely and comfortably.

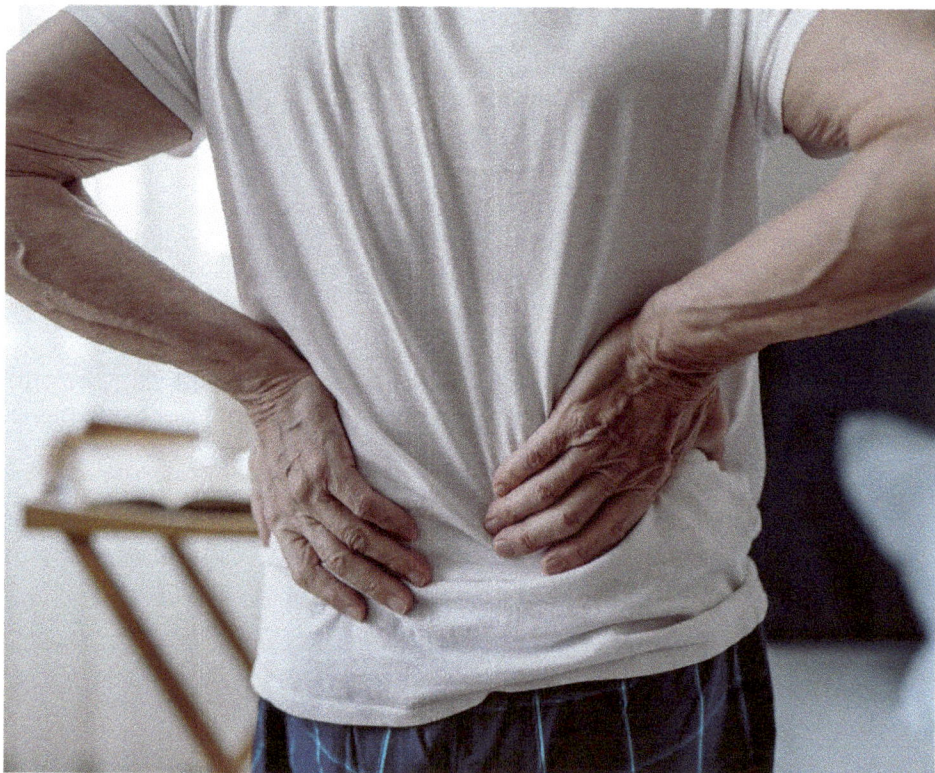

QUESTIONS ABOUT NECESSARY PROVIDED ASSISTANCE FOR BACK PAIN SUFFERERES

These questions focus on practical strategies for obtaining the necessary assistance and adjusting at work to manage or prevent back pain effectively.

HOW CAN I TALK TO MY EMPLOYER OR HR DEPARTMENT ABOUT MY BACK PAIN AND THE NEED FOR ACCOMMODATIONS?

Whether or not to avoid sexual activity during the acute phase of back pain depends on several factors, including the severity of your pain, the specific nature of your back injury, and how your body responds to movement. Here are some considerations to help you make an informed decision:

Prepare for the Conversation:
*   Understand Your Rights: Familiarise yourself with your company's policies on accommodations and your rights under laws like the Americans with Disabilities Act (ADA) in the U.S., which protects employees with medical conditions.

*   Know What You Need: Before speaking to your employer, clearly identify the accommodations that would help you manage your back pain. These might include ergonomic adjustments, flexible work hours, more frequent breaks, or the ability to work from home.

*   Gather Documentation: If possible, obtain a letter or documentation from your healthcare provider outlining your condition and the recommended accommodations. This can help support your request and provide clarity on your needs.

Request a Meeting:

- Schedule a Private Meeting: Request a private meeting with your manager or HR representative to discuss your situation. Avoid discussing personal medical issues in an open or informal setting.

- Choose the Right Time: Find a time when you can have an uninterrupted conversation, allowing both you and your employer to focus on the discussion.

Communicate Clearly and Professionally:

- Explain Your Condition: Start by briefly explaining your back pain and how it affects your ability to work. You don't need to go into great detail about your medical history but focus on how it impacts your job performance.

  Example: "I've been experiencing significant back pain, which has been affecting my ability to sit for long periods and complete my tasks comfortably."

- Focus on Solutions: Emphasise that you're looking for ways to maintain your productivity and continue contributing to the team, with some adjustments to help manage your condition.

  Example: "To continue performing my job effectively, I believe some accommodations would help, such as an ergonomic chair, a standing desk, or the ability to take short breaks to stretch."

- Be Specific About Your Needs: Clearly outline the accommodations you're requesting and explain how they would help you manage your back pain while maintaining your work responsibilities.

  Example: "I would like to request an ergonomic assessment of my workspace and the possibility of adjusting my work hours to include more breaks."

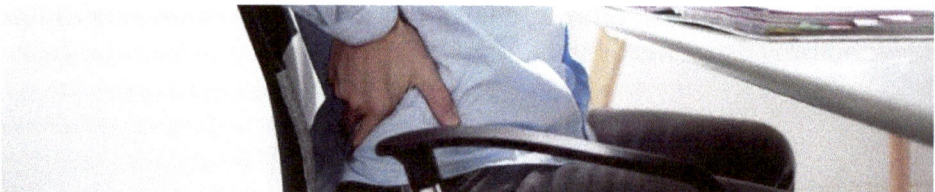

Be Open to Discussion:

- Invite Feedback: Ask your employer or HR representative for their thoughts on your request and be open to discussing practical solutions.

   Example: *"I'm open to discussing what accommodations are feasible and how we can work together to find the best solution."*

- Discuss Alternatives: If your initial request isn't possible, be prepared to discuss alternative solutions that could also help manage your condition.

Follow Up in Writing:

- Document the Conversation: After your meeting, follow up with a written summary of what was discussed and agreed upon. This helps ensure that everyone is on the same page and provides a record of the conversation.

   Example: *"Thank you for meeting with me to discuss accommodations for my back pain. As we discussed, I'll be using an ergonomic chair and taking more frequent breaks to manage my condition. Please let me know if there's anything else I should be aware of."*

Monitor and Adjust as Needed:

- Evaluate the Effectiveness: Once accommodations are in place, assess whether they are helping manage your back pain effectively. If not, don't hesitate to request further adjustments.

- Keep the Lines of Communication Open: Stay in touch with your employer or HR department about how the accommodations are working and any changes in your condition.

Know When to Escalate:

- If You Face Resistance: If your request for accommodations is not being taken seriously or if you face discrimination, consider seeking advice from a legal professional or your union (if applicable). You can also file a complaint with the Equal Employment Opportunity Commission (EEOC) in the U.S. if you believe your rights are being violated.

Approaching your employer or HR department about your back pain and the need for accommodations involves clear communication, preparation, and a focus on finding solutions that allow you to perform your job effectively while managing your condition. By being proactive and professional, you can help ensure that your needs are met and that you're able to work comfortably and safely.

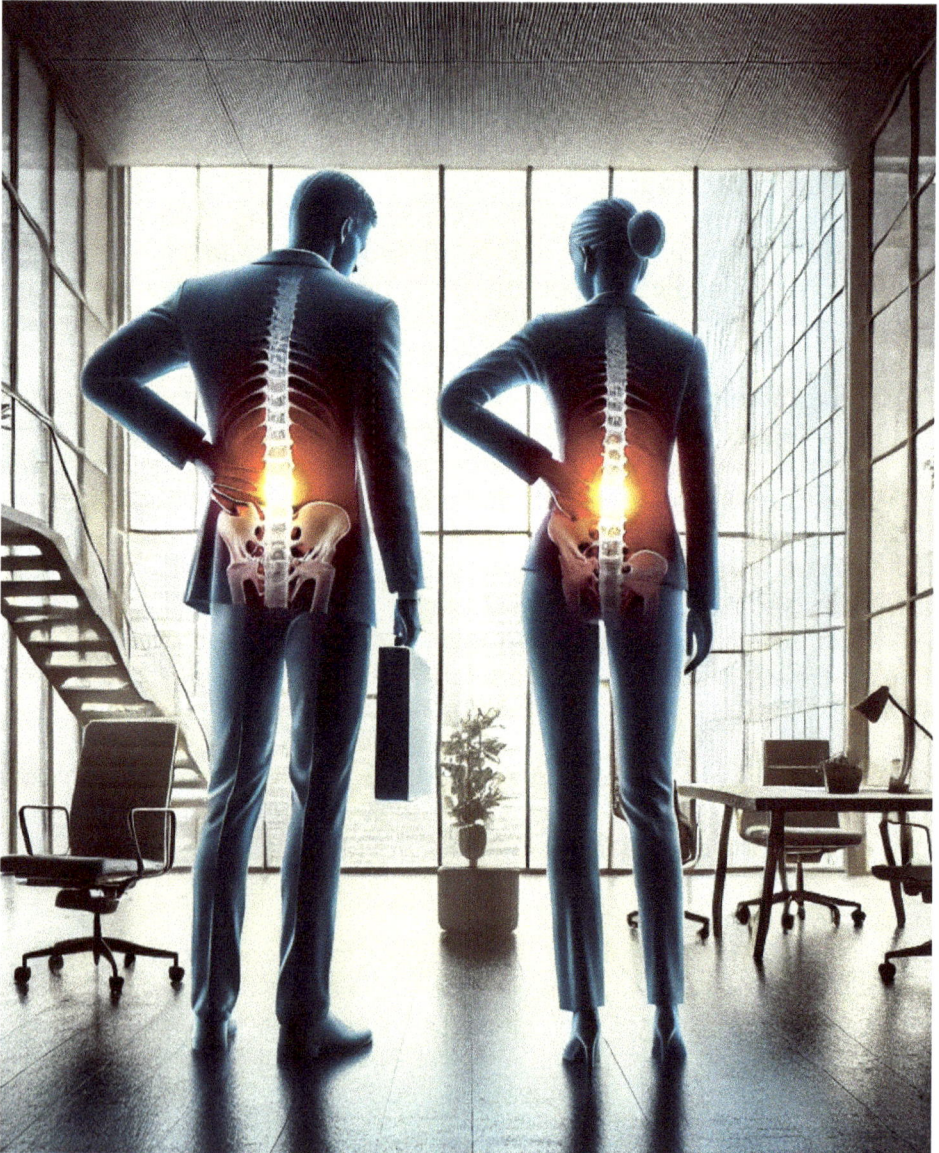

ARE THERE SPECIFIC TASKS OR DUTIES I SHOULD AVOID AT WORK TO PREVENT WORSENING MY BACK PAIN?

To prevent worsening your back pain at work, it's important to identify and avoid tasks or duties that place undue strain on your back. Here are specific tasks and activities you should consider modifying or avoiding:

Heavy Lifting and Carrying:
- Avoid Lifting Heavy Objects: Lifting heavy items can strain your back muscles and increase the risk of injury, especially if done improperly.

- Use Proper Lifting Techniques: If lifting is unavoidable, bend at your knees and hips, keep the object close to your body, and avoid twisting your torso. Use your legs to lift, not your back.

- Request Assistance: If you need to move heavy objects, ask for help from a colleague or use mechanical aids like a dolly or cart.

Prolonged Sitting or Standing:
- Avoid Long Periods of Sitting: Sitting for extended periods, especially in a non-ergonomic chair, can increase pressure on your lower back.

- Take Frequent Breaks: If your job requires long periods of sitting, take breaks every 20-30 minutes to stand, stretch, and walk around. Adjust your chair and desk setup to support good posture.

- Avoid Prolonged Standing: Standing for long periods without moving can also strain your back. If your job involves standing, try to shift your weight frequently, use a footrest, and wear supportive footwear

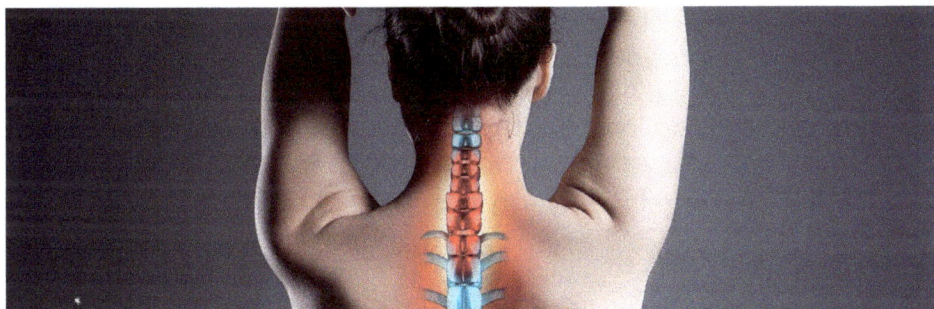

Repetitive Movements:
- Avoid Repetitive Bending or Twisting: Tasks that involve repetitive bending, twisting, or reaching can aggravate back pain by stressing your spine and muscles.

- Modify Your Workstation: Arrange your workstation so that commonly used items are within easy reach to minimise unnecessary movements.

- Use Ergonomic Tools: Consider using ergonomic tools and equipment that reduce the need for repetitive motions or awkward postures.

Pushing, Pulling, or Dragging Objects:
- Avoid Forceful Movements: Pushing, pulling, or dragging heavy objects can strain your back muscles and joints.

- Use Mechanical Aids: Whenever possible, use carts, trolleys, or other mechanical aids to move heavy items. If you must push or pull something, use both hands, keep your back straight, and engage your core muscles

Working in Awkward Postures:
- Avoid Awkward or Unbalanced Postures: Tasks that require you to work in awkward positions, such as reaching overhead, leaning forward, or working on your knees, can strain your back.

- Adjust Your Work Environment: Make ergonomic adjustments to your workstation or tools to avoid awkward postures. For example, use a step stool to reach high shelves instead of overstretching.

High-Impact Activities:
- Avoid High-Impact Tasks: Tasks that involve jumping, running, or other high-impact activities can exacerbate back pain by placing sudden stress on your spine.

- Request Modifications: If your job involves high-impact activities, discuss with your employer about modifying these tasks to reduce the impact on your back.

Stressful Tasks:
- Avoid High-Stress Situations: High-stress tasks can contribute to muscle tension, including in your back, which may worsen pain.

- Manage Stress: Practice stress management techniques, such as deep breathing, mindfulness, or taking short breaks, to help reduce the impact of stress on your back pain.

Inadequate Workstation Setup:
- Avoid Non-Ergonomic Workstations: A poorly set-up workstation can contribute to poor posture, leading to back pain. Ensure your chair, desk, and computer monitor are positioned to support a neutral spine.

- Request Ergonomic Adjustments: Work with your employer or HR department to adjust your workstation ergonomically. This may include adjusting your chair height, using a footrest, or positioning your monitor at eye level.

To prevent worsening your back pain at work, avoid tasks that involve heavy lifting, prolonged sitting or standing, repetitive movements, and awkward postures. Prioritise ergonomic adjustments, take frequent breaks, and use mechanical aids when necessary. If certain tasks are unavoidable, discuss accommodations with your employer to help manage your condition while maintaining your work responsibilities.

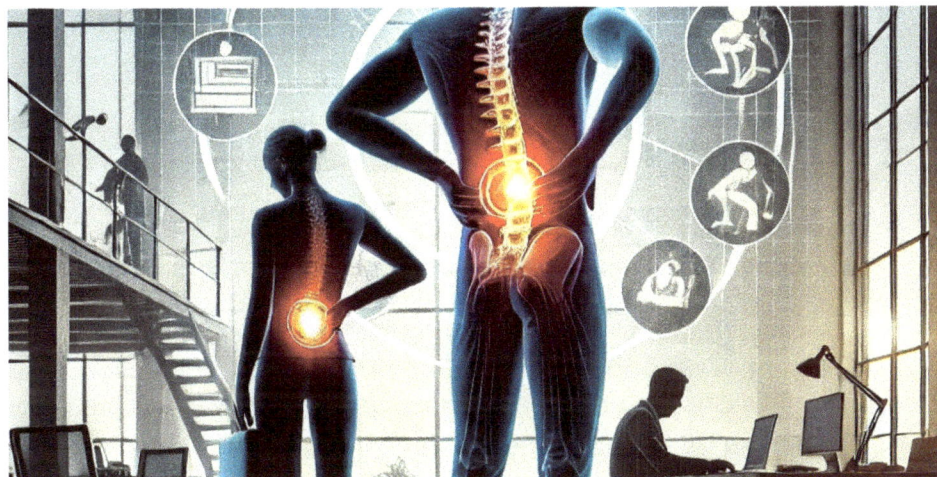

HOW OFTEN SHOULD I TAKE BREAKS TO STRETCH OR MOVE AROUND TO MANAGE MY BACK PAIN AT WORK?

Taking regular breaks to stretch and move around is crucial for managing back pain at work. Here's a guideline on how often you should take these breaks:

Frequency of Breaks:
- Every 20-30 Minutes: Aim to take a short break every 20-30 minutes, especially if you are sitting or standing for prolonged periods. This helps prevent stiffness, improves circulation, and reduces the strain on your back.

- Microbreaks: These are brief breaks lasting 1-2 minutes where you can stand up, stretch, or walk around. They can be incorporated frequently throughout the day.

- Hourly Breaks: In addition to microbreaks, take a slightly longer break (5-10 minutes) every hour to move around, stretch more thoroughly, and change your posture.

What to Do During Breaks:
- Stretching: Perform gentle stretches targeting your back, neck, shoulders, and legs. Simple stretches like the ones mentioned below can help alleviate tension:

  - Shoulder Shrugs and Rolls: Gently shrug your shoulders up towards your ears and then roll them back and down.

  - Seated Forward Bend: While seated, gently bend forward to reach for your toes, keeping your back straight to stretch your lower back.

  - Neck Stretch: Tilt your head to one side, bringing your ear towards your shoulder, and hold for 15-20 seconds on each side.

- Movement: Walk around your office, do a quick lap around your floor, or simply stand and march in place for a minute. Movement helps reduce stiffness and promotes circulation.

- Posture Check: Use your break to reset your posture. Ensure your feet are flat on the floor, your back is straight, and your shoulders are relaxed.

Use of Ergonomics:
- Adjust Workstation: Take these breaks as an opportunity to adjust your workstation setup. Ensure your chair, desk, and computer monitor are positioned to maintain a neutral spine.

- Alternate Between Sitting and Standing: If possible, alternate between sitting and standing throughout the day. Consider using a sit-stand desk to change positions without disrupting your work.

Use Reminders:
- Set Timers: Use a timer or reminder on your phone or computer to prompt you to take breaks. There are also apps designed to remind you to move and stretch at regular intervals.

- Incorporate Breaks into Routine: Integrate these breaks naturally into your workflow. For example, stand up whenever you take a phone call, or stretch while reading emails.

Taking regular breaks to stretch and move around every 20-30 minutes, along with longer hourly breaks, is essential for managing back pain at work. These breaks help prevent stiffness, reduce strain on your back, and improve circulation. By incorporating stretches, posture checks, and movement into your routine, you can better manage your back pain and maintain your productivity throughout the workday.

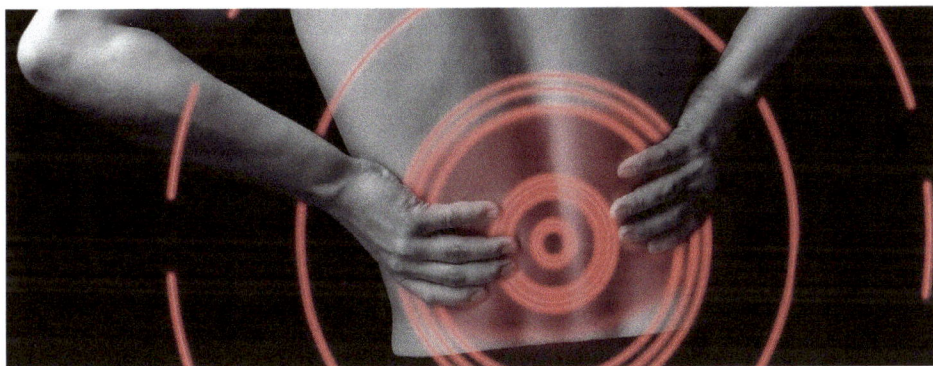

CAN I REQUEST A STANDING DESK, AND HOW DO I USE IT PROPERLY TO AVOID BACK PAIN?

You can certainly request a standing desk as part of your workplace accommodations to help manage back pain. Standing desks can reduce the strain associated with prolonged sitting, but it's important to use them correctly to avoid creating new issues. Here's how to go about requesting one and how to use it properly:

How to Request a Standing Desk:
- Review Company Policies: Check if your company has a policy for ergonomic accommodations. Many companies are open to providing standing desks, especially if it's supported by a healthcare provider's recommendation.

- Prepare Your Request: When requesting a standing desk, explain how it will help you manage your back pain and improve your productivity. Mention any recommendations from your doctor or physical therapist.

   Example: *"I've been experiencing back pain that's exacerbated by prolonged sitting. I believe a standing desk could help me manage my pain more effectively and maintain my productivity."*

- Discuss with HR or Your Manager: Schedule a meeting with your HR department or manager to discuss your request. Be prepared to provide documentation from your healthcare provider if necessary.

How to Use a Standing Desk Properly:
- Alternate Between Sitting and Standing: It's important not to stand all day. Alternate between sitting and standing throughout the day to reduce strain on your back and legs. Aim for a 1:1 or 2:1 ratio of sitting to standing.

   Example: *Stand for 20-30 minutes, then sit for 30-60 minutes, and repeat.*

- Maintain Proper Posture: Whether standing or sitting, keep your posture in check:

    - Standing: Stand with your feet shoulder-width apart, weight evenly distributed, knees slightly bent and avoid locking your knees. Keep your head aligned with your spine and your shoulders relaxed.

    - Sitting: When sitting, your feet should be flat on the floor, your back supported by the chair, and your knees at a 90-degree angle.

- Adjust Desk Height: Your desk should be at elbow height when standing, allowing your forearms to rest comfortably on the desk at a 90-degree angle. The top of your monitor should be at or slightly below eye level to avoid straining your neck.

- Use a Footrest or Anti-Fatigue Mat: Consider using a footrest to shift your weight periodically or an anti-fatigue mat to reduce strain on your feet and legs while standing.

- Wear Supportive Footwear: Wear comfortable, supportive shoes that provide good arch support. Avoid standing in high heels or flat shoes with poor support.

- Move Frequently: Even when standing, it's important to shift your weight, change your stance, and move around periodically. You can also do small stretches or march in place to keep your muscles engaged.

Additional Tips for Using a Standing Desk:
- Start Gradually: If you're new to using a standing desk, start by standing for short periods and gradually increase the duration as your body adjusts.

- Monitor Your Body's Response: Pay attention to how your body feels while using the standing desk. If you notice any discomfort in your back, legs, or feet, adjust your setup or reduce your standing time.

- Incorporate Ergonomic Accessories: Use accessories like monitor arms, keyboard trays, and adjustable chairs to optimise your standing desk setup.

Requesting a standing desk is a reasonable accommodation for managing back pain and using it correctly can help reduce strain and improve comfort. By alternating between sitting and standing, maintaining proper posture, and making necessary ergonomic adjustments, you can use a standing desk effectively to support your back health at work.

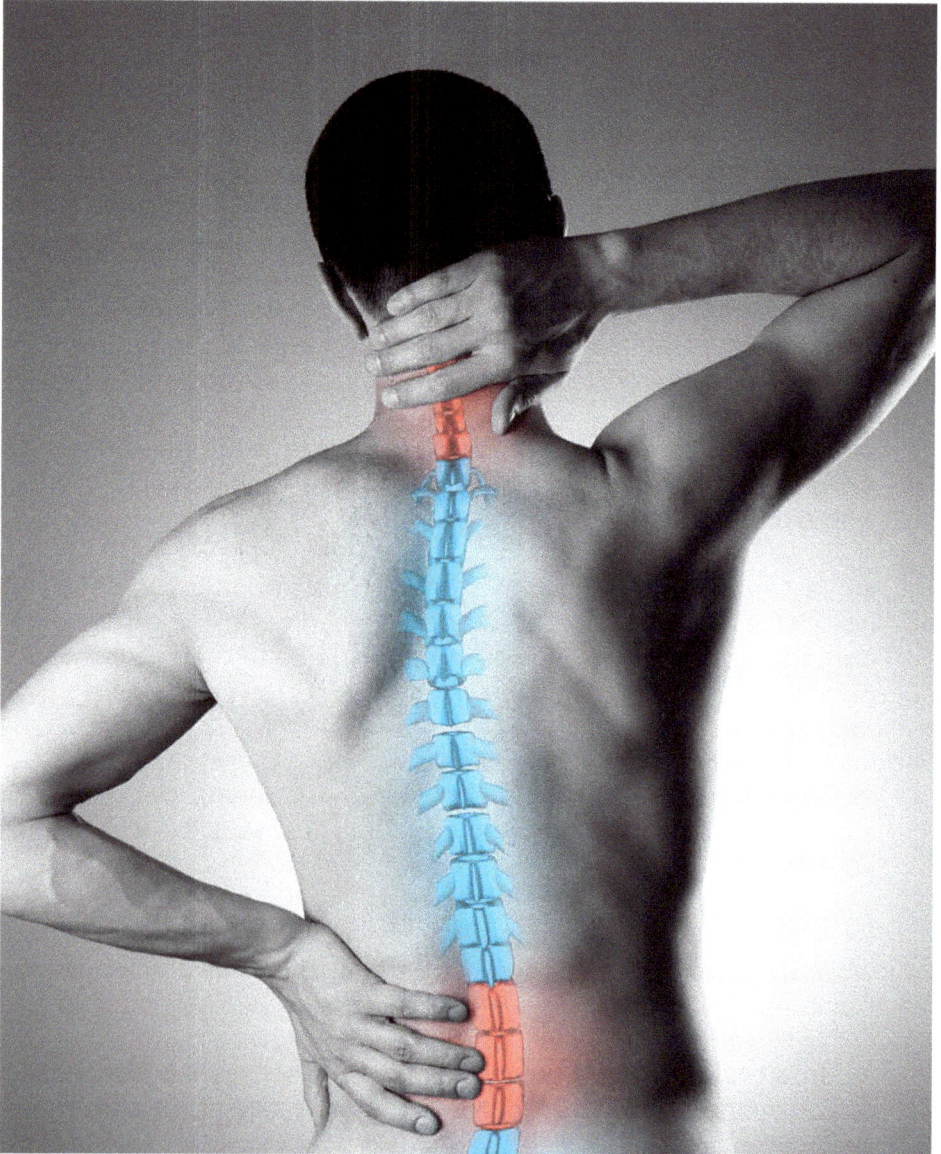

IS THERE SPECIAL EQUIPMENT OR TOOLS I CAN USE TO REDUCE STRAIN ON MY BACK WHILE PERFORMING MY JOB?

There are several types of special equipment and tools that you can use to reduce strain on your back while performing your job. These tools are designed to promote better posture, support your back, and make tasks more ergonomically friendly. Here are some options:

Ergonomic Chairs

Features to Look For: Adjustable height, lumbar support, armrests, and a swivel base. The chair should allow you to keep your feet flat on the floor, with your knees at a 90-degree angle and your back supported.

Benefits: A good ergonomic chair helps maintain the natural curve of your spine and reduces the risk of slouching, which can strain your lower back.

Standing Desks and Sit-Stand Workstations

Adjustable Desks: Allows you to switch between sitting and standing throughout the day, reducing the strain associated with prolonged sitting.

Benefits: Helps to reduce pressure on the lower back, improve circulation, and encourage movement.

Footrests

Adjustable Footrests: Provide support for your feet if they don't comfortably reach the floor when sitting. A footrest can help maintain proper posture and reduce strain on your lower back.

Benefits: Helps maintain a neutral spine position and can reduce pressure on the lower back.

Lumbar Support Cushions

Memory Foam Cushions: These cushions are designed to support the natural curve of your lower back, providing additional support while sitting.

Benefits: Reduces pressure on the lower spine and helps maintain proper posture throughout the day.

Monitor Arms or Stands

Adjustable Monitor Arms: These allow you to position your computer monitor at eye level, reducing the need to hunch over or tilt your head down.

Benefits: Promotes a neutral neck position and reduces strain on the upper back and shoulders.

Keyboard Trays

Ergonomic Keyboard Trays: These trays can be adjusted for height and tilt, allowing you to keep your wrists in a neutral position while typing.

Benefits: Reduces strain on the wrists, shoulders, and upper back by promoting a more ergonomic typing posture.

Anti-Fatigue Mats

Standing Mats: Used when standing for extended periods, these mats provide cushioning and support to reduce pressure on your feet, legs, and lower back.

Benefits: Helps reduce fatigue and discomfort in the lower body, promoting better posture and less strain on the back.

Ergonomic Tools for Lifting and Carrying

Lifting Aids: Devices like lifting belts, dollies, or carts can help you move heavy objects without straining your back.

Proper Techniques: Using these tools, combined with proper lifting techniques (bending at the knees, not the back), can significantly reduce the risk of back injury.

Adjustable Desks and Workstations

Sit-Stand Workstations: These allow you to alternate between sitting and standing, helping to reduce the strain of prolonged sitting, or standing.

Benefits: Encourages movement and allows you to maintain better posture throughout the day.

Wearable Posture Correctors

Posture Braces: These are wearable devices that gently pull your shoulders back to prevent slouching, which can contribute to back pain.

Benefits: Helps to maintain proper posture throughout the day, reducing strain on the back and shoulders.

Document Holders

Adjustable Document Holders: Keep your documents at eye level next to your monitor, so you don't have to look down repeatedly, reducing neck and upper back strain.

Benefits: Promotes a neutral head position and reduces strain on the neck and upper back.

Supportive Footwear

Orthotic Insoles: These can provide additional arch support and cushioning if you're on your feet a lot.

Supportive Shoes: Shoes with good arch support and cushioning can reduce strain on your lower back, especially if your job involves standing or walking.

Using special equipment and tools like ergonomic chairs, standing desks, footrests, lumbar cushions, and lifting aids can significantly reduce strain on your back while performing your job. These tools, combined with proper ergonomics and posture, can help you manage back pain more effectively and prevent further strain or injury. Consider discussing these options with your employer or HR department to create a more ergonomic workspace that supports your back health.

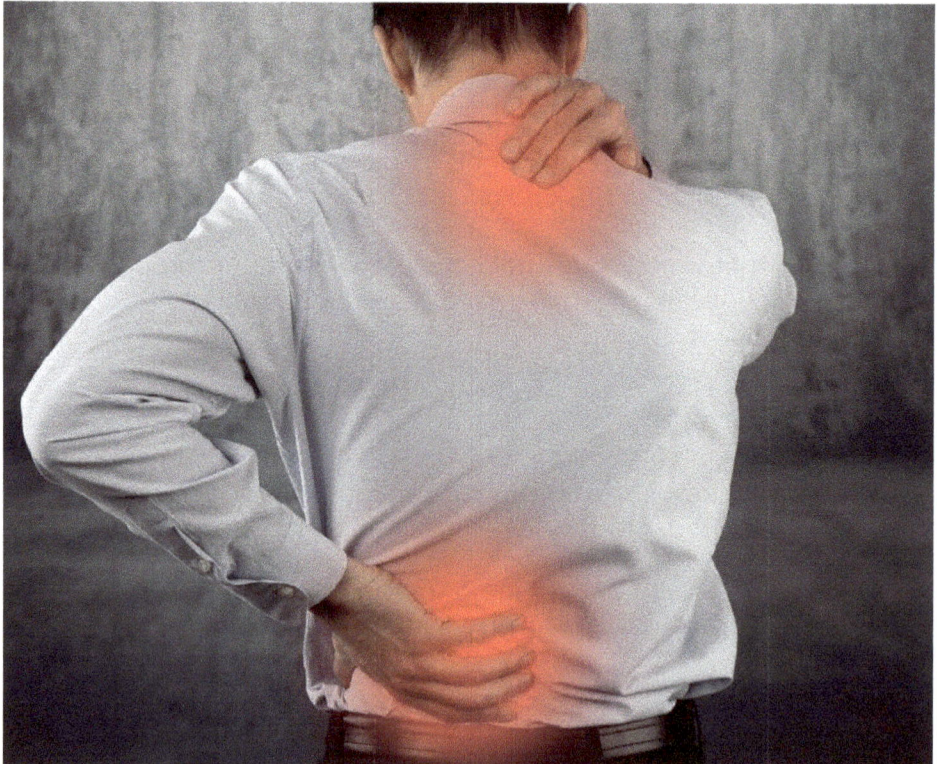

WHAT EXERCISES OR STRETCHES CAN I DO AT MY WORKSTATION TO HELP RELIEVE BACK PAIN?

Incorporating exercises and stretches at your workstation can help relieve back pain by reducing muscle tension, improving circulation, and promoting better posture. Here are some effective exercises and stretches you can do without leaving your desk:

Seated Forward Bend:
How to Do It:
- Sit on the edge of your chair with your feet flat on the floor, hip-width apart.

- Slowly bend forward from your hips, reaching your hands towards your feet or the floor.

- Let your head and neck relax and hold the position for 15-30 seconds.

- Slowly roll back up to a seated position

Benefits: Stretches the lower back, hamstrings, and relieves tension in the spine.

Seated Spinal Twist:
How to Do It:
- Sit up straight in your chair with your feet flat on the floor.

- Place your right hand on the back of your chair and your left hand on your right knee.

- Gently twist your torso to the right, looking over your shoulder.

- Hold for 15-30 seconds, then switch sides.

Benefits: Improves spinal mobility, stretches the upper and lower back, and relieves tension.

Shoulder Shrugs:

How to Do It:

- Sit or stand with your arms relaxed at your sides.

- Inhale deeply and lift your shoulders up towards your ears.

- Hold for a few seconds, then exhale and drop your shoulders back down.

- Repeat 10 times.

Benefits: Relieves tension in the shoulders and upper back, promotes relaxation.

Seated Cat-Cow Stretch:

How to Do It:

- Sit on the edge of your chair with your feet flat on the floor and hands on your knees.

- As you inhale, arch your back, and lift your chest, looking slightly upward (Cow Pose).

- As you exhale, round your back and tuck your chin to your chest (Cat Pose).

- Repeat this movement 5-10 times, moving slowly and with your breath.

Benefits: Increases spinal flexibility, relieves lower back tension, and improves posture.

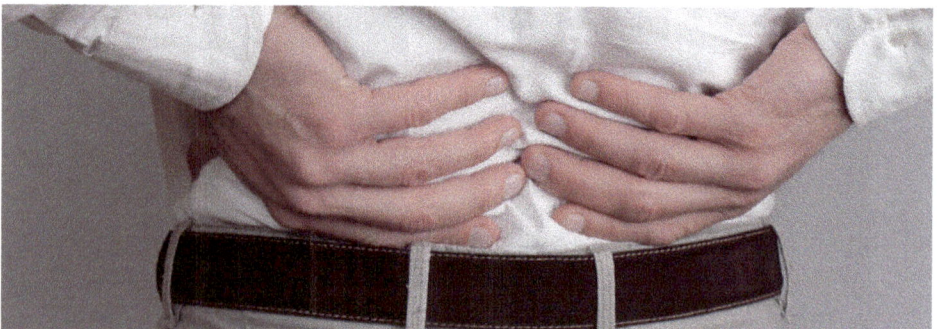

Upper Back Stretch:
How to Do It:
- Sit up straight with your feet flat on the floor.

- Extend your arms straight in front of you, with your palms facing each other.

- Clasp your hands together and gently push your hands forward, rounding your upper back.

- Hold for 15-30 seconds, then release.

Benefits: Stretches the upper back and shoulders, relieves tension between the shoulder blades.

Neck Stretch:
How to Do It:
- Sit or stand with your back straight.

- Gently tilt your head to one side, bringing your ear towards your shoulder.

- Hold for 15-30 seconds, then switch sides.

- For a deeper stretch, place your hand on the side of your head and apply gentle pressure.

Benefits: Stretches the neck muscles, reduces tension, and alleviates upper back pain.

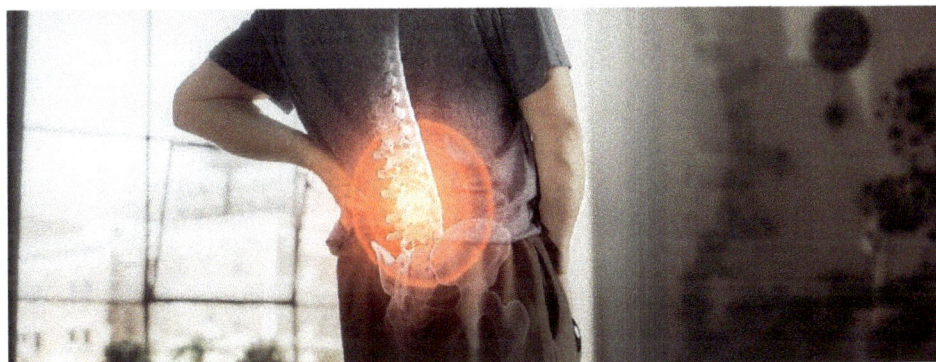

Seated Hip Stretch:
How to Do It:
- Sit on the edge of your chair with your feet flat on the floor.

- Cross your right ankle over your left knee, forming a figure four with your legs.

- Gently press down on your right knee while leaning forward slightly from your hips.

- Hold for 15-30 seconds, then switch sides.

Benefits: Stretches the hips and lower back, which can help relieve lower back pain.

Standing Hamstring Stretch:
How to Do It:
- Stand up and place one foot on a low chair or desk, keeping your leg straight.

- Lean forward slightly from your hips, reaching towards your toes.

- Hold for 15-30 seconds, then switch legs.

Benefits: Stretches the hamstrings and lower back, which can reduce tension in the lower back.

Seated Pelvic Tilt:
How to Do It:
- Sit on the edge of your chair with your feet flat on the floor.

- Tilt your pelvis forward, arching your lower back slightly.

- Then tilt your pelvis backward, flattening your lower back.

- Repeat this movement 10 times, focusing on the movement in your lower back.

Benefits: Strengthens the lower back and core, improves posture, and reduces back stiffness.

Wrist and Forearm Stretch:
How to Do It:
- Extend one arm straight out in front of you, palm facing down.

- Use your other hand to gently pull back on the fingers of the extended hand, stretching the wrist and forearm.

- Hold for 15-30 seconds, then switch sides.

Benefits: Reduces tension in the wrists and forearms, which can help prevent strain from typing.

Tips for Incorporating These Exercises:

- Set Reminders: Use a timer or reminder app to prompt you to stretch every 30 minutes to an hour.

- Breathe Deeply: Focus on deep, slow breathing during each stretch to enhance relaxation and muscle release.

- Stay Consistent: Make these stretches a regular part of your workday routine to prevent and manage back pain effectively.

Incorporating these exercises and stretches into your workday routine can help relieve back pain, improve flexibility, and reduce muscle tension. These simple movements can be done at your workstation, allowing you to manage your back health while staying productive.

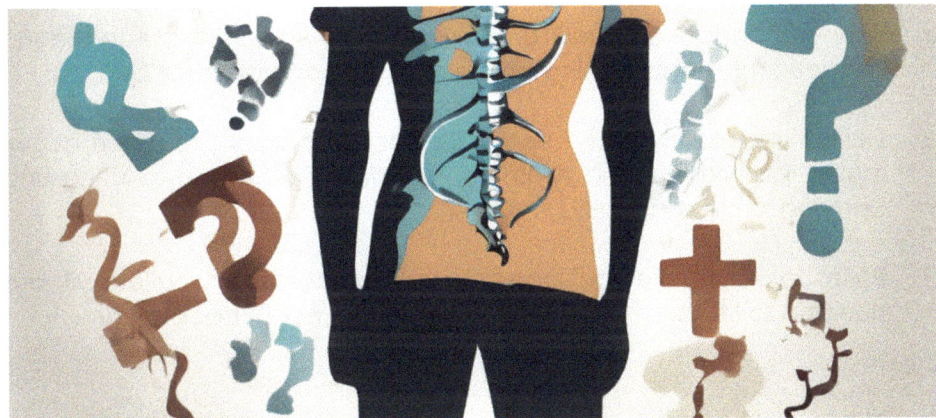

WHAT EQUIPMENT NEED TO ASK FOR A HAULAGE COMPANY TO PROVIDE ME IF I SUFFER FROM LOW BACK PAIN?

If you suffer from low back pain and work for a haulage company, it's important to request specific equipment and tools that can help reduce strain on your back and prevent further injury. Here are some items you should consider asking for:

Ergonomic Seat and Lumbar Support:
- Ergonomic Truck Seat: Request a truck seat that provides good lumbar support, adjustable seat height, and seat angle. An ergonomic seat can help maintain proper posture during long driving hours and reduce pressure on your lower back.

- Lumbar Support Cushion: If a new seat is not an option, ask for a lumbar support cushion that you can place on your existing seat to help support the natural curve of your lower back.

Vehicle Modifications and Adjustments:
- Adjustable Steering Wheel: Ensure the truck has an adjustable steering wheel that allows you to maintain a comfortable and neutral arm position without straining your back.

- Proper Mirror Placement: Adjust mirrors so you can see clearly without having to twist or turn excessively, which can strain your back.

Lifting Aids:
- Powered Liftgate: Request a truck with a powered liftgate to reduce the need for manual lifting of heavy items from the truck bed.

- Dollies and Hand Trucks: Use dollies or hand trucks to move heavy loads. This reduces the strain on your back compared to lifting and carrying items manually.

- Pallet Jacks: A pallet jack can be used to move heavy pallets without needing to lift them manually, reducing the risk of back injury.

Tools that Secure the Load:
- Load Bars and Straps: Use load bars and ratchet straps to secure loads properly. This prevents items from shifting during transport, reducing the risk of having to move heavy items repeatedly.

- Automated Tie-Down Systems: If available, request automated or easier-to-use tie-down systems to minimise the physical effort required to secure loads.

Anti-Fatigue Mats:
- Standing Mats: If you spend time standing on hard surfaces while loading or unloading, request anti-fatigue mats to stand on. These mats reduce pressure on your feet, legs, and lower back.

Supportive Footwear:
- Safety Shoes with Good Arch Support: Request or ensure that you are provided with safety shoes that have good arch support and cushioning. Proper footwear is essential in reducing the impact on your lower back when standing or walking on hard surfaces.

Hydraulic or Electric Lifting Equipment:
- Hydraulic Tail Lifts: If you frequently load and unload heavy items, hydraulic tail lifts can help minimise the need for manual lifting.

- Electric Hoists: Electric hoists can be used to lift heavy items, reducing the risk of back injury from lifting or awkward movements.

Back Support Belt:
- Lifting Belt or Back Support Belt: While not a substitute for proper lifting techniques, a back support belt can provide additional stability and support during lifting tasks.

Ergonomic Workstation for Paperwork:
- Adjustable Desk: If you spend time doing paperwork or using a computer in the truck or office, request an adjustable desk or workstation that allows you to work comfortably without straining your back.

- Document Holders: Use document holders to position paperwork at eye level, reducing the need to hunch over.

Training on Proper Lifting Techniques:

- Lifting Technique Training: Request training on proper lifting techniques and ergonomics to help prevent back injuries. Understanding how to lift correctly can significantly reduce the risk of injury.

Requesting the right equipment and tools from your haulage company is crucial for managing low back pain and preventing further injury. Be proactive in communicating your needs to your employer, and make sure you use the equipment correctly to minimise strain on your back. Proper ergonomic support, lifting aids, and training can make a significant difference in maintaining your back health while performing your job duties.

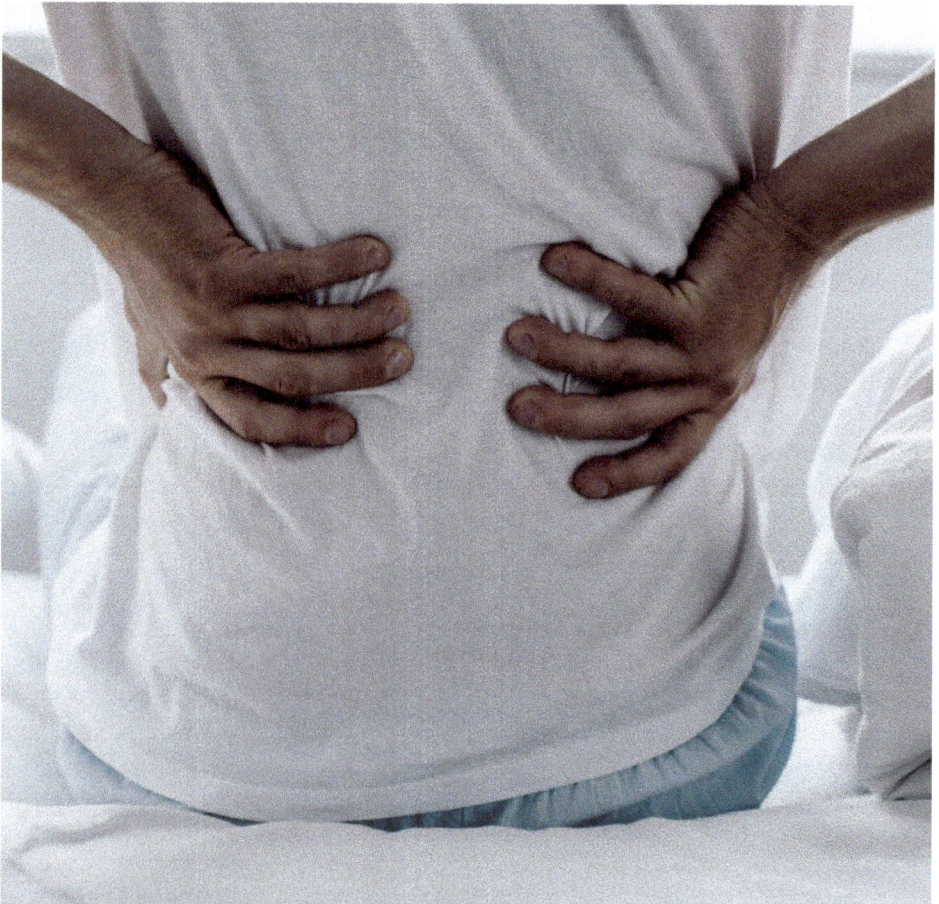

HOW CAN I ENSURE MY WORKSTATION IS SET UP CORRECTLY TO MINIMISE BACK STRAIN?

Setting up your workstation correctly is essential to minimise back strain and promote good posture throughout your workday. Here are some key steps to ensure your workstation is ergonomically optimised:

Chair Setup:
- Adjustable Height: Your chair should be at a height where your feet rest flat on the floor, and your knees are at a 90-degree angle. Your thighs should be parallel to the ground.

- Lumbar Support: Ensure your chair has proper lumbar support to maintain the natural curve of your lower spine. If your chair lacks built-in lumbar support, consider using a lumbar cushion.

- Seat Depth: The seat should allow about 2-3 inches of space between the back of your knees and the edge of the seat. If necessary, adjust the seat depth or use a cushion to achieve this.

- Armrests: Adjust the armrests so that your shoulders are relaxed, and your elbows are at a 90-degree angle when typing. Your forearms should be parallel to the ground.

Desk and Monitor Positioning:
- Desk Height: Your desk should be at a height that allows your forearms to be parallel to the floor when typing, with your elbows at a 90-degree angle. If your desk is too high, consider using a footrest; if it's too low, consider raising it.

- Monitor Height: The top of your monitor should be at or slightly below eye level, so you don't have to tilt your head up or down. The screen should be about an arm's length away from your face.

- Monitor Position: Position the monitor directly in front of you to avoid twisting your neck. If you use multiple monitors, place the primary one directly in front of you and the secondary one to the side.

Keyboard and Mouse Placement:

- Keyboard Position: Place your keyboard so that it's directly in front of you, with your wrists in a neutral position (not bent up or down) while typing. The keyboard should be at a height that allows your elbows to be at a 90-degree angle.

- Mouse Placement: Keep your mouse close to your keyboard to minimise reaching. Your mouse should be at the same height as your keyboard, and your wrist should remain neutral while using it.

- Wrist Support: Consider using a wrist rest or gel pad to keep your wrists in a neutral position and reduce strain.

Foot Position:

- Flat on the Floor: Ensure your feet are flat on the floor or on a footrest. Avoid crossing your legs, as this can lead to uneven weight distribution and strain on your lower back.

- Footrest: If your feet don't reach the floor comfortably, use a footrest to provide support and maintain a 90-degree angle at your knees.

Lighting and Screen Glare:

- Reduce Glare: Position your monitor to avoid glare from windows or overhead lights. Consider using an anti-glare screen if needed.

- Proper Lighting: Ensure your workspace is well-lit to reduce eye strain. Use task lighting if necessary to illuminate your work area without creating glare on your screen.

Workstation Organisation:

- Keep Items Within Reach: Arrange frequently used items, such as your phone, notepad, and other tools, within easy reach to avoid unnecessary stretching or twisting.

- Document Holder: If you work with documents, use a document holder positioned next to your monitor at eye level to avoid looking down frequently.

Take Regular Breaks:

- Microbreaks: Take short breaks every 20-30 minutes to stand, stretch, and move around. This helps reduce muscle fatigue and prevents stiffness.

- Position Changes: Alternate between sitting and standing if possible, using a sit-stand desk or simply standing up during phone calls or meetings.

Proper Posture:

- Neutral Spine: Maintain a neutral spine posture, with your back straight, shoulders relaxed, and ears aligned with your shoulders.

- Avoid Slouching: Be mindful of slouching or leaning forward, as this can strain your lower back.

Ergonomic Accessories:

Consider Ergonomic Tools: If needed, invest in ergonomic accessories like a standing desk, an adjustable keyboard tray, or an ergonomic chair to further support your posture and comfort.

Setting up your workstation to minimise back strain involves adjusting your chair, desk, monitor, keyboard, and other accessories to support good posture and reduce strain on your back. Regularly assess your workstation setup and adjust as needed to ensure it continues to meet your ergonomic needs. Taking frequent breaks and practicing good posture are also essential for maintaining back health throughout the workday.

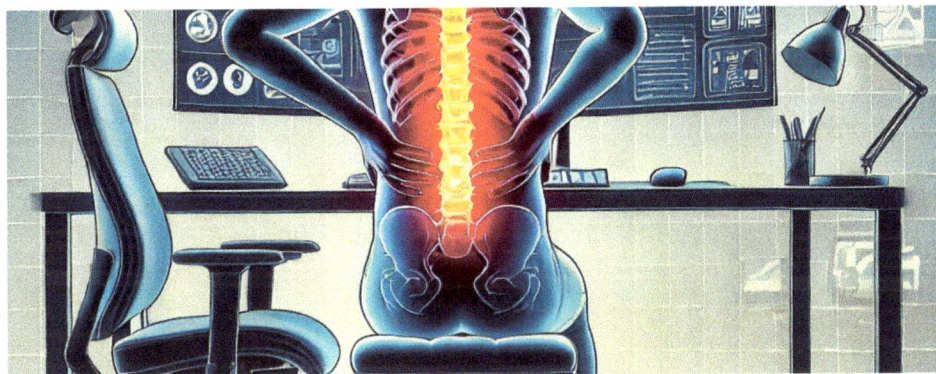

IF MY JOB INVOLVES HEAVY LIFTING OR PHYSICAL LABOUR, WHAT TECHNIQUES OR SUPPORT CAN I USE TO PROTECT MY BACK?

If your job involves heavy lifting or physical labour, it's crucial to use proper techniques and supportive equipment to protect your back and prevent injury. Here are key strategies to help you lift safely and reduce the risk of back pain:

Proper Lifting Techniques:

- Plan the Lift: Before lifting, assess the load to determine its weight and stability. Plan your route and ensure the path is clear of obstacles.

- Bend at the Knees, Not the Waist: Squat down by bending at your knees and hips, keeping your back straight. Avoid bending at the waist, as this puts excessive strain on your lower back.

- Keep the Load Close to Your Body: Hold the object as close to your body as possible to reduce the leverage on your back. Keeping the load close to your centre of gravity helps maintain balance and reduces strain.

- Lift with Your Legs: Use the strength of your leg muscles to lift the load, not your back. As you lift, straighten your legs while keeping your back straight.

- Avoid Twisting: Keep your feet pointed in the direction you're moving to avoid twisting your spine. If you need to turn, pivot with your feet instead of twisting your torso.

- Maintain a Neutral Spine: Keep your back straight and maintain the natural curve of your spine throughout the lift. Avoid rounding your back.

- Use Smooth Movements: Lift the load smoothly and avoid jerky or sudden movements, which can strain your back.

Supportive Equipment:

- Lifting Belts: A lifting belt can provide additional support to your lower back by increasing intra-abdominal pressure, which helps stabilise your spine. However, lifting belts should be used as an adjunct to proper lifting techniques, not a substitute.

- Mechanical Aids: Use tools like dollies, hand trucks, pallet jacks, or forklifts to move heavy loads whenever possible. These tools reduce the need for manual lifting and can significantly decrease the risk of back injury.

- Back Supports or Braces: In some cases, wearing a back support or brace can provide additional stability and remind you to maintain good posture. However, these should not replace proper lifting techniques.

- Assistive Lifting Devices: Use assistive devices like hoists or cranes for particularly heavy or awkward loads. These devices take on the weight, reducing the physical strain on your body.

Workplace Ergonomics:

- Height-Adjustable Workstations: If your job involves repetitive lifting, a height-adjustable workstation can help position loads at an optimal height to minimise bending and lifting.

- Proper Tool Placement: Organise tools and materials within easy reach to minimise unnecessary bending, stretching, or lifting.

- Team Lifting: For heavy or bulky items, use a team lift. Coordinate with your coworkers to lift and carry the load together, distributing the weight evenly.

Physical Conditioning:

- Strengthen Core Muscles: Regularly engage in exercises that strengthen your core muscles, including your lower back, abdominals, and hips. A strong core provides better support for your spine during lifting activities.

- Flexibility Training: Incorporate flexibility exercises, such as stretching and yoga, to maintain good mobility in your back, hips, and legs. Flexible muscles are less prone to injury.

- Cardiovascular Fitness: Maintain overall cardiovascular fitness to improve endurance and reduce fatigue during physical labour.

Breaks and Rest:
- Take Regular Breaks: Give your muscles time to recover by taking regular breaks during physically demanding tasks. This can help prevent overuse injuries.

- Pace Yourself: Avoid rushing through tasks that require heavy lifting or repetitive motions. Work at a steady pace to reduce the risk of straining your back.

Education and Training:
- Lifting Training: Participate in workplace training programs that teach proper lifting techniques and the use of ergonomic tools. This training can provide valuable knowledge to protect your back.

- Safety Awareness: Stay aware of your surroundings and potential hazards. Take the time to assess each situation and use the appropriate technique or tool for the job.

Protecting your back when performing heavy lifting or physical labour involves using proper lifting techniques, supportive equipment, and maintaining good physical conditioning. By following these guidelines and using available resources, you can minimise the risk of back injury and ensure a safer working environment. If you're unsure about the best practices for your specific job, consult with a safety officer or ergonomic specialist for personalised advice.

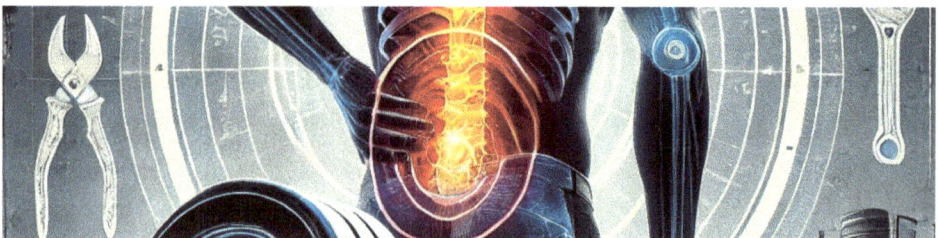

EPILOGUE

Closing the final part of this journey through the questions and answers surrounding low back pain, it is clear that this condition is not just a physical ailment but a complex experience that touches every aspect of life. From the frustration of finding the right diagnosis to the challenges of daily living, each question posed, and each answer given has been a step toward understanding, managing, and, living with low back pain.

This book was born out of a need to address the myriad concerns that those suffering from low back pain face every day. It is not just a compilation of medical facts and advice but a testament to the resilience and determination of individuals who refuse to be defined by their pain. The questions, you have asked, reflect a deep desire to regain control, to find relief, and to lead fulfilling lives despite the challenges of living with chronic pain.

The answers provided, which in some cases are repeated between the different chapters, while grounded in medical knowledge, are also infused with empathy, and understanding. They recognise that each person's experience with low back pain is unique, and that what works for one may not work for another.

This is why this book does not offer a one size fits all solution but rather a collection of insights, strategies, and options that you can explore and tailor to your own needs.

As you close this book, remember that the journey does not end here. Managing low back pain is an ongoing process that requires patience, persistence, and a willingness to adapt. It is about finding what works for you, staying informed, and most importantly, advocating for your health and well-being.

Let this book serve as a companion on your path, a resource you can return to whenever you need guidance or reassurance. Whether you are seeking to understand your condition better, looking for new ways to manage your symptoms, or simply needing to know that you are not alone, the answers you find here are meant to empower you.

To everyone who is living with low back pain, and chronic pain, know that your questions matter, and that finding the right answers is a crucial part of your journey to health. May this book be a beacon of hope, a source of comfort, and a reminder that while low back pain may be a part of your life, it does not have to define it.

Increase your knowledge and fight for knowledge and management of your low back pain. Stay healthy, strong, and keep up for brighter days ahead. Ask constantly as this way you continue to learn, and knowledge is power.

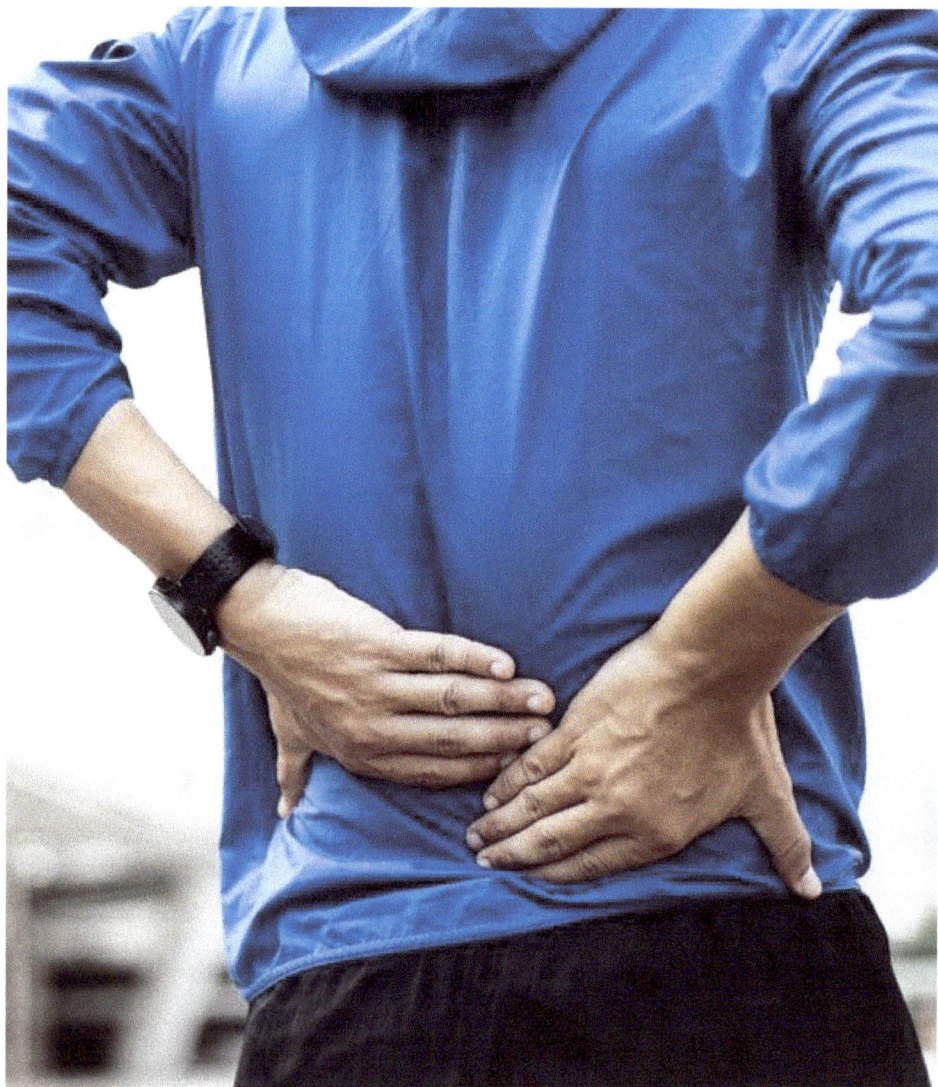

FURTHER NOTICE

More information on any of these subjects you can find in the following books written by the Author:

1. **PAIN MANAGEMENT FOR CHRONIC LOW BACK PAIN SUFFERERS**
   https://amzn.eu/d/06GUFWVP

2. **KAMA SUTRA FOR BACK PAIN SUFFERERS**
   https://amzn.eu/d/0fVMV3RO

3. **FROM BACK PAIN TO PRODUCTIVITY:**
   A Business Leader's Guide Supporting Employees
   https://amzn.eu/d/0iLoRnl5

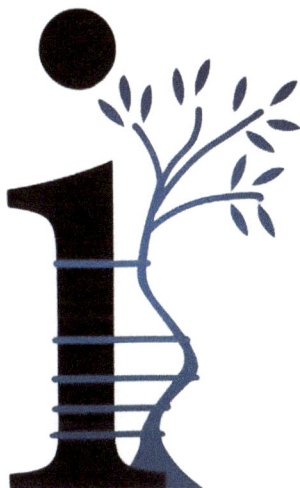

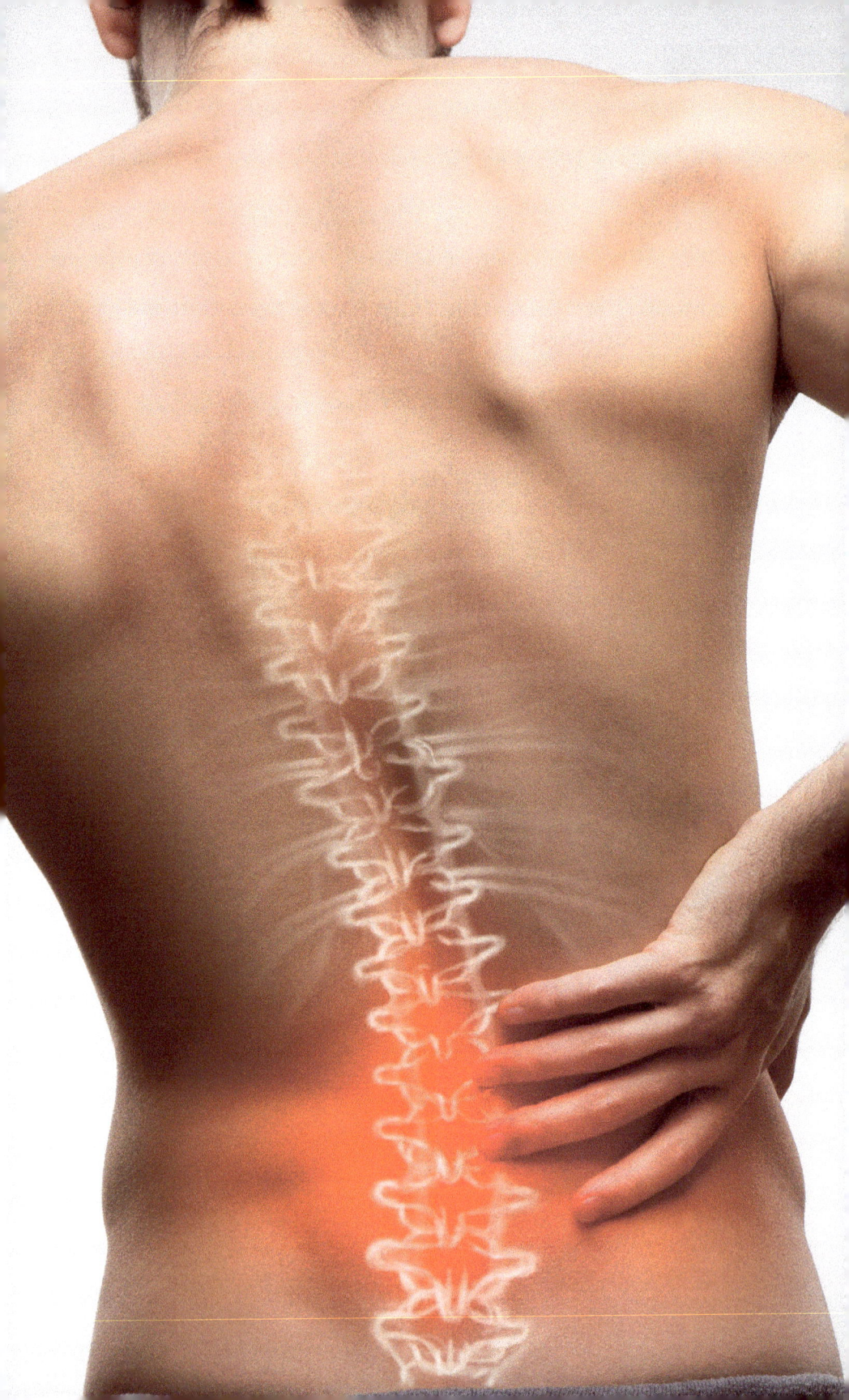

.

9 781068 673771